An Irish guide to goo

Ch...up
Children

Edited by
Siobhán Cleary

in association with

**TOWN
HOUSE**

Published in 1994 by
Town House and Country House
Trinity House
Charleston Road
Ranelagh, Dublin 6
Ireland
in association with RTE

A CIP catalogue record for this book is available from the British
Library.

ISBN: 0-948524-88-X

Cover photo of Siobhán Cleary by Frank Fennell Photography
Typeset by Typeform Repro, Dublin.
Printed in Ireland by Colour Books Ltd, Dublin

CONTENTS

Siobhán Cleary has a background in theatre and teaching. She began her career as a journalist writing newspaper features and reporting on the *Gay Byrne Show,* and she has been presenter of *Check Up* since it began. She also produces educational videos for medicine and dentistry and she lectures in communication skills at the School of Dental Science, Trinity College, Dublin. She is married to theatre director Joe Dowling and they have two teenage children.

FOREWORD

Check Up, RTE's health programme, is now in the seventh year of its very successful run. Its great popularity has always been due to its concentration on the experience of ordinary people who have had the misfortune at some stage of their lives to become patients.

One would think that if someone is ill and in pain, the last thing they need is a television crew in their livingroom asking them how they feel. But we have invariably found that the opposite is the case, and we never cease to be impressed by the willingness of people to expose their own pain and fear in order to help others who may be going through the same ordeal.

This is particularly so when it comes to children and their parents. There is perhaps no greater anxiety than that which is caused by a sick child, and this makes it all the more difficult to talk about it publicly on a television programme. But it also makes it all the more valuable when parents do share their often heart-rending experiences with a wider audience, and this has always been the motivation of those parents who have allowed us into their homes and their lives at a time of great trial to themselves and their families.

This puts a great responsibility on us as a programme to deal as sensitively and unobtrusively as we can with everyone who has had the selflessness to publicly expose their most private anxieties, pain, fears and sometimes, tragically, their grief. It is a responsibility that we take very seriously indeed, and the programme operates on the premise that it is the people we interview who have complete control over what is said and what is omitted. This factor has been critical to the success of *Check Up* throughout its existence.

We would like to express our deep gratitude to all those who over the years have spoken of their experiences on *Check Up.* Without their generosity and selflessness, there would never have been a *Check Up* in the first place.

Mary Raftery
Series Producer
Check Up

INTRODUCTION

Bringing up children can be the most rewarding job in the world, but it can also be fraught with anxieties, as children often seem to go from one bout of sickness to another in rapid succession. Their tendency to develop an illness very quickly can be quite alarming, and their ability to bounce back swiftly to good health can be equally astonishing.

As the first 'Check Up' book, *The Check Up Guide to Good Health*, began to take shape, I soon realised that there was also a need for an Irish health book devoted entirely to children's health. *Check Up Children* has the same aim as its predecessor, that of debunking many of the myths and removing many of the fears that surround health and medicine. Its authors are all distinguished experts, many of whom have appeared on the *Check Up* programme. They offer parents clear explanations about the common childhood conditions, and give practical advice on how best to help children recover at home, and when medical help should be sought.

The subjects included cover a wide range of ages, from the newborn baby up to the adolescent. To avoid using the unwieldy term 'he/she', in each alternate chapter the child is referred to as either 'he' or 'she'.

It can be useful for future reference to have a record of your child's illnesses, treatments and immunisations, but as the years go by, it is easy to forget the details, particularly when you have more than one child. I have included a Health Record Chart at the back of the book that you can photocopy for each child.

I would like to thank all the writers for their co-operation and dedication, and for taking such care in making complex ideas very accessible. Thank you also to publisher Treasa Coady of Town House and copy-editor Elaine Campion for their enormous contribution to this book.

In remembering my own childhood I thank my parents Nancy and Frank, who made it almost a pleasure to be ill in bed for a few days. A special thanks to my children Susanna and Ronan for giving me first-hand experience in childcare, and to my husband Joe for sharing the nursing and comforting.

I would like to express my appreciation to all my colleagues on *Check Up* for their support over the last six years, including those who are currently with the programme: Mary Raftery, the series producer, reporters Mary O'Sullivan and John Murray, and production assistants Hilary Courtney and Una McHenry.

Over the years *Check Up* has featured many children who have suffered conditions ranging from the very minor to the chronic and life-threatening. Each one has shown enormous strength and courage in coping with discomfort and pain, but sadly some like Niamh and Eoin Maguire have lost their long battle with illness. I would like to dedicate the book to all those children and their parents.

Siobhán Cleary

A HEALTHY PREGNANCY

DR PETER BOYLAN

It is not so long since pregnancy was regarded as a time of confinement, when a woman hid herself away from society, lay on a couch as often as possible, and started 'eating for two'. Today's pregnant woman is much more active. She is likely to be working full time, inside or outside the home, and enjoying most of the sporting activities and exercise she always did.

According to obstetrician Dr Peter Boylan, who is Master of the National Maternity Hospital, the vast majority of women who become pregnant are likely to have a healthy baby at the end of their nine months, and Ireland now may be the safest place in the world in which to have a baby.

A healthy pregnancy is one that ends with a healthy mother and a healthy baby. In modern Ireland the majority of pregnancies that progress beyond twelve weeks have a successful outcome. The caveat 'progress beyond twelve weeks' is because approximately 15 per cent of diagnosed pregnancies end in miscarriage in the first twelve weeks. The chances of miscarriage decline markedly after that.

Most women are in excellent general health at the beginning of pregnancy and, in the absence of a pre-existing condition such as diabetes, are equally healthy after the birth of their child. While pregnancy can have many effects, both physical and psychological, that may make a woman feel 'unwell', most are attributable to the pregnancy and few cause any long-term problems for the majority of women.

The death of a mother due to a complication of pregnancy is rare in Ireland; indeed Ireland has the lowest rate of maternal mortality in the industrialised world, better than any of the European Union countries, Scandinavia, or the United States of America.

Statistics for Irish babies are equally reassuring. More than 90 per cent of babies who reach 500gm (1.2lb) birth weight, and who are normally formed, will survive; handicap in the form of cerebral palsy and/or mental handicap is also rare and affects approximately two per 1000 children in all western societies where figures are available.

These statistics represent the hard facts of pregnancy outcome for women in Ireland today, but there is more to a healthy pregnancy than figures, however comforting they may be.

A HEALTHY MOTHER

The reproductive years, from teens to mid forties, are usually a woman's healthiest. Sixty per cent of births are to mothers between the ages of twenty-five and thirty-four, and a further 30 per cent are included by extending the age range from twenty to forty. Only 10 per cent of births therefore occur at the extremes of the reproductive age group.

In an ideal world, all pregnancies would occur in women who are physically fit, eat a balanced diet, are immunised against German measles, and have a positive psychological approach to pregnancy and childbirth. Preparation therefore begins well before conception.

Body changes in pregnancy

Pregnancy produces dramatic changes in a woman's body. Conception stimulates the production of several hormones, which affect different parts of the body.

- There is a dramatic increase in blood volume, of approximately 40 per cent, which begins as early as four weeks after conception and partly explains the bloated feeling that is characteristic of early pregnancy; the muscle-relaxing effects of one of the hormones, progesterone, is another contributory factor.

- Frequent urination is another symptom of early pregnancy, again caused by the blood volume increase; the kidneys take time to adapt to the change in work-load.

- Constipation is a common feature of pregnancy and is a direct result of the muscle-relaxing properties of pregnancy hormones. Because iron preparations can exacerbate this problem, many doctors do not prescribe iron supplements until well into pregnancy, when a woman has become used to the changes in her body.

- Fatigue, similar to jet lag, is a common feature in the first few months.

- Many people suffer some degree of nausea and vomiting during pregnancy. The cause is not known but it is unusual for it to persist beyond twelve weeks. On occasions it may be so severe as to warrant hospital admission. Vomiting, no matter how severe or prolonged, has no effect on the developing foetus.

- Heartburn is caused by acid regurgitation. Normally, acid secretions are kept in the stomach by a valve-like muscle at the stomach entrance. In pregnancy, this muscle relaxes and allows acid regurgitation/heartburn to occur.

- Headaches are common during pregnancy and are probably due to the increased blood volume causing stretching of the blood vessels in the head.

- Vaginal secretions increase during pregnancy, probably as a protective mechanism to prevent infection ascending into the uterus (womb).

- Crampy pains in the lower abdomen are not unusual, and are of no consequence unless they are accompanied by bleeding, or are severe and prolonged.

- Some women suffer from nosebleeds, and again this may be a consequence of the increased blood volume and resultant nasal congestion.

- Varicose veins are uncommon in a first pregnancy, but may occur in subsequent pregnancies. Support stockings will relieve the symptoms, which usually go away after delivery.

- Haemorrhoids (piles) are another form of varicose vein, and are associated with constipation. They may also result in occasional episodes of bleeding.

This daunting catalogue of minor ailments might be enough to put even the most stoic off pregnancy. But many women will go through the entire nine months with none of these problems, and it is rare to find someone who suffers from all of them. Most are intermittent in nature and virtually all resolve themselves without treatment after the baby is born.

Maintaining health and fitness

There is only a limited amount a woman can do to avoid these irritations of pregnancy.

- No drugs, even those available over the counter, should be taken without consulting your doctor.

- A healthy diet, high in fibre, with plenty of fluids, will lessen the chances of constipation, haemorrhoids and stomach cramps, quite apart from improving general health.

- Small frequent meals, avoiding spicy foods and taking antacids (such as Rennies, Maalox, etc) all help to minimise heartburn and nausea.

- A reasonable amount of exercise — swimming seems to be especially beneficial — improves general health and will help to build up the fitness and stamina that may be needed later on when it comes to the hard physical work of labour. Walking, tennis and golf are all harmless during pregnancy and may be continued as long as comfort permits. Aerobic classes may be continued, but the more vigorous exercises should be avoided. One of the hormones of pregnancy, relaxin, softens the ligaments that keep our joints in place. Excessive stretching may strain joints that would normally be unaffected. Occasionally in late pregnancy, women will experience a sharp knife-like stabbing pain in the vagina; this is due to the rubbing together of the two pubic bones at the front of the pelvis as a result of relaxin having softened the ligaments that normally keep them tightly bound together.

- Low back pain due to the strain of carrying the developing baby may be eased by adapting a straight-back posture, sleeping on a hard bed, and perhaps the application of mild heat, such as a hot water bottle.

- Weight gain should be restricted to less than 13kg (2 stone) for the entire pregnancy. This is important from the mother's, rather than the baby's, point of view. Early in pregnancy there may be significant weight gain, usually because of fluid retention. Women who suffer a lot of vomiting may lose weight, but can be reassured that this won't harm the developing baby. Keeping your weight under control is a matter of diet and exercise, and is easier said than done because of the effect of pregnancy itself. If weight gain exceeds 13kg it becomes progressively more difficult to lose weight after birth.

- There is no medical reason why you shouldn't have sexual intercourse during pregnancy, although nausea and fatigue in the first three months, and physical difficulties in the last three months may be impediments.

THE OLDER MOTHER

In obstetrics, a woman is described as older if she is thirty-five years or more when she conceives. From the woman's point of view the description is quite inaccurate, as pregnancy itself presents no danger to the mother as long as complications, which can occur at any age, don't develop. While some complications such as high blood pressure occur more frequently in older women, they are by no means inevitable, and age by itself is not a reason for not getting pregnant. The age at which a woman conceives is largely a matter of individual choice, but it must be remembered that natural fertility declines with advancing age. The decline appears to be gradual until a woman enters her forties, and is very steep after that age. Many women now postpone childbearing until their thirties, and they should be reassured that, as long as their general health is good, pregnancy should present no challenge beyond the ordinary.

The only risk with advancing age in pregnancy is that the baby has an increased chance of having a chromosomal problem, particularly Down's Syndrome. This risk is probably a lot lower than most people imagine; it is less than 1 per cent until the age of forty, and at the age of forty-five it is 1 in 32. It is not until a woman is forty-seven or forty-eight years of age that there is a 10 per cent risk that her baby will have Down's Syndrome. Other rare chromosome problems show a small increase with advancing age. These figures should be further reassurance about the likely normal outcome of pregnancy, regardless of the mother's age.

PREPARATION FOR LABOUR

Antenatal classes are advisable for the first-time mother, and many women who have already had a baby derive great benefit from refresher classes. Preparatory classes for pregnancy and labour assist the mother in choosing the right diet and deciding on the right amount of exercise, and help to dispel many of the myths of pregnancy — which are legion! Relaxation techniques that are particularly beneficial during labour are an important feature of the classes. Preparation for labour improves the chances of a normal birth and therefore helps towards a speedy recovery.

A HEALTHY BABY

We all began life when our parent's egg and sperm met, joined together in fertilisation, and divided their genetic material on a roughly 50/50 basis to create a new individual. Enclosed in a protective, fluid-filled sac, foetal development proceeds at a rapid pace, so that by fourteen weeks all the body organs are formed. Subtle changes take place during the rest of pregnancy, but the most vulnerable time is the first few weeks.

A mother's healthy lifestyle assists normal foetal development, but does not guarantee it. A counsel of perfection would be to avoid alcohol completely, eat only wholesome foods, take a moderate amount of exercise, and get plenty of rest and sleep.

There is no evidence that an occasional drink does any harm to a developing baby, although alcohol does cross into the baby's bloodstream, and if the mother has a glass of wine so too does the baby. Studies have shown that a single measure of spirits taken in the middle of pregnancy sedates the baby in the same way that it depresses an adult's brain. Many women find that they lose their taste for alcohol early in pregnancy, and this may well be a natural mechanism to protect the developing embryo from harm. No responsible parent feeds alcohol to their children, so perhaps the American attitude of no alcohol at all during pregnancy is correct. Nevertheless, the warm brandy and sugar our mothers gave us in infancy to soothe us when agitated is unlikely to have caused permanent damage. As with most things, moderation is wise. Heavy drinking, on the other hand, may cause foetal alcohol syndrome — a collection of physical and developmental abnormalities that may be associated with learning disabilities. This is thankfully a rare condition, which only occurs in cases where the mother has been drinking heavily during pregnancy.

Smoking is harmful to both the mother and her baby, and from the baby's point of view it is the ultimate example of passive smoking. It may slow the baby's growth by reducing her supply of food and oxygen. While statistics have shown an association between smoking and miscarriage, it is wrong to place all the blame on smoking, as this may well induce an unwarranted feeling of guilt on top of an already fraught situation. Pregnancy presents an incentive to stop smoking and is an opportunity that should be grasped eagerly.

There is now evidence that a 5mg tablet of Folic Acid, if taken daily around the time of conception and in the very early stages of pregnancy, may help in preventing the congenital (from birth) defect of spina bifida.

THE USE OF ULTRASOUND

Ultrasound is a diagnostic technique in which a two-dimensional image is created by passing high-frequency sound waves into the body. This technology has revolutionised obstetric care and is one of the greatest advances in medicine this century. Ultrasound scans have almost become a routine part of antenatal care in western countries. Advances in ultrasound technology have provided a window into the uterus, which shows the exact position of the foetus and the placenta (afterbirth). This means that blood samples may be taken from the umbilical cord for a variety of diagnostic tests, and blood transfusions may be given directly to the foetus in cases of severe Rhesus disease.

There is no evidence, however, that routine scanning benefits the baby, and indeed a recent study from Australia suggested that repeated scans might slow the growth of the baby. However, a single scan does not appear to cause any problems whatsoever, and many couples find that a view of their baby at sixteen to twenty weeks is a very rewarding, and reassuring, experience. A scan done at this time confirms when the baby may be expected to arrive, whether it is a single or multiple pregnancy, and will usually show if there is a major problem. It is very important to understand, however, that many problems will not be apparent on a scan. Later in pregnancy a scan may be done if, for example, it is suspected that growth is slow, or if the mother is bleeding. If a pregnancy goes overdue, many doctors will recommend a scan to check the condition of the baby, and particularly the fluid surrounding the baby, to see if induction of labour is medically required.

BIRTH

A healthy birth is where labour starts spontaneously, progresses normally, and delivery is a result of the mother's efforts, with a minimum of intervention. Indeed, the quality of care may be judged by the rate of intervention in the form of forceps and Caesarean delivery. As a general rule anything above 10 per cent for either is probably too high. In Ireland the rate of Caesarean section is approximately 10 per cent, but in the United States it is more than double at 23 per cent, and is a source of great concern to patients and doctors alike. One of the reasons quoted for the high rate in the United States is the fear doctors have of being sued by their patients if something goes wrong during a natural delivery.

On a first birth it is not unusual for the mother either to have a tear at the vagina, or to require a cut (episiotomy) in the course of delivery; this occurs less frequently on subsequent births.

Labour is well named, as it is hard work for the mother, so it is advisable to be well prepared physically for the event. Recovery from birth is quicker among those who have a normal delivery and who do not require stitches. Antenatal classes go a long way towards minimising anxiety, and this helps the woman cope with the physical and psychological stresses of labour.

———————————————

Dr Peter Boylan MAO, FRCPI, FRCOG is Master of the National Maternity Hospital, Holles Street, Dublin 2.

ACCIDENTS AND EMERGENCIES

DR ROISÍN HEALY

Accidents are the commonest cause of death in childhood after the age of nine months. The majority of fatalities are caused by road traffic accidents, followed by fire, drownings, inhalation and suffocation. But fatal accidents are only the tip of the iceberg, and many more children are injured. About 10 to 15 per cent of these have some permanent problem as a result of their injuries. Many children are also injured in accidents inside the home, especially younger children. Dr Roisín Healy, Accident and Emergency Consultant at Our Lady's Hospital, Crumlin, describes how easily accidents can happen, and gives practical advice on how we can make the environment safer for our children, and what to do when an emergency occurs.

CHILD DEVELOPMENT AND ACCIDENTS

The types of accident children have are intimately linked to their physical, intellectual and social development and growth. This is best illustrated by examples:

Physical development

A newborn baby can fall only if dropped, or if the person carrying him falls. Within a few months, however, he can wriggle and begin to turn, and is capable of rolling off a bed. Later, when he is able to crawl, he may tumble down the stairs.

Intellectual development

A toddler may scald himself with a hot drink as he has not yet developed the concept of 'hot' being dangerous. Similarly, a five-year-old cannot judge the speed of oncoming cars, though he can understand the concept of 'hot'.

Social behaviour and growth

Older children love to play and explore — they climb, they run out onto the road after a ball or cross the road to a friend. They are thinking of their game, not of its dangers.

Children must be understood on their own terms. It is not true to say that children's behaviour is unpredictable. What *is* true is that adults do not always understand the predictability of children's behaviour. It is quite predictable that a five-year-old will concentrate on the game at hand and will run out onto the road after a ball. Most fatal road traffic accidents involving children as pedestrians are caused by young male drivers who have not yet had experience of rearing children of their own. Adults need to be educated in accident prevention and in making the environment safe for their children.

MAKING THE HOME SAFE

Because young children spend so much time in the home, this is the commonest place for the under-fives to be injured. As children get older and more mobile and begin to play outdoors, road traffic accidents and school accidents increase, but the home still remains a dangerous place.

Most accidents in the home occur in the kitchen, the livingroom and the hallway. I would recommend that all couples buying their first family home should 'borrow' a toddler to bring along to any showhouse they may visit. They will soon be aware of how 'child friendly' the house really is.

Kitchen

In the kitchen, a child is at risk from many different sources. He may burn himself on a hot object such as a saucepan, scald himself by pulling the flex of a boiling kettle, poison himself by getting into household cleaning agents or medicine stored in accessible cupboards. Look around your kitchen and pretend that you are a two-year-old. A bubbling saucepan or a shining hot iron looks very attractive but will burn a little hand put up to touch it.

There are a number of simple things you can do to help make your kitchen safer. Put saucepans well back on the cooker. Buy a cordless kettle and use the minimal amount of cord from the socket to the base, and store it well back on the counter-top. Use safety catches on all cupboard doors. Don't leave pointed objects such as scissors lying around. If you get rid of an old fridge, make sure you take off the door before discarding it so that a child cannot climb into it, close the door on himself and smother. It is wise to have a fire-blanket and a small fire-extinguisher in the home, preferably hanging in clear view in the kitchen.

Hall and stairs

You should never have glass panelling on internal doors of the house, particularly in areas where children run, play and slam doors. Every year many accidents occur that involve glass-panelled doors, as well as windows with larger sheets of glass. If you live in a house that has doors like this, get the glass changed to safety glass or, better still, change the doors. If there is glass panelling at the bottom of the stairway, which a child may hit if he slides or falls down the stairs, make sure it is safety glass.

Check the banisters of your stairs for any horizontal bars that a child could climb through. Bars should be vertical, and the width between them should be no more than 10cm (4in). If a child falls through the banisters he is likely to suffer a skull fracture or worse. It is preferable to have stairs that are either L-shaped or U-shaped so that there is a shorter distance to fall.

When an infant begins to crawl it is advisable to put gates at the top and bottom of the stairs. Badly fitting carpet or carpet with holes on which children might trip should either be got rid of or made safe. Toys, etc. shouldn't be left lying around, either on the steps of the stairs or in the hallway where people might slip.

Make sure you have a smoke alarm in the hall and another on the landing area.

Livingroom/playroom

In the livingroom or play area, there should be no sharp objects such as edges of fire surrounds or corners of tables where children may knock against them. All toys and sharp objects that may be of danger to the exploring toddler, such as small pieces of Lego, should be stored safely. Older brothers and sisters should be taught to be caring in protecting younger children against such dangers. Electrical sockets should be positioned where they won't form an attraction for the exploring toddler. This can be done, for example, by putting a heavy piece of furniture in front of them. Avoid trailing flexes and extension cords where children may trip over them. Store matches in a secure place, preferably in a location unknown to the children, as even older children like to experiment with fire, particularly if their parents are absent. Always use safety fireguards that have sides and tops.

Safety glass should be used in doors and windows, particularly those at a low level. As a temporary measure polyester plastic film (safety film) can be fitted over existing glass; although this is not as satisfactory as laminated glass, it does reduce flying glass fragments, but there may be problems with cleaning and it may scratch. It is safer to board up a high-risk area of glass than to have a child scarred for life. All large areas of glass should be well marked to prevent children crashing through them by mistake. The risks of such collisions may be lessened by putting obstacles such as plant pots or furniture in front of the glass.

Bathroom

Scalds from hot water are a constant danger. Make sure you have a thermostat fitted, set to a maximum of $54^{\circ}C$ ($130^{\circ}F$). Thermostatically controlled mixer taps are also an excellent idea. Young children must never be left unattended in the bath. They can drown, even in a few inches of water.

Bedrooms

If you use bunk-beds remember there is inevitably some hazard involved in putting a small child to sleep four or five feet up in the air. No child under the age of six years should be in an upper bunk. Make sure that the bunk-bed you buy has two full safety rails, one at each side of the top bunk, as you might not always put the bunk against a wall. No bunk-bed should have a gap in the base or bed-head of more than 7.5cm (3in). In Britain, it is now illegal to sell new or secondhand bunks with gaps wider than this. Bunks should not have any fittings that can be undone without using a tool. Any ladder or foothold must be firmly secured. There should be at least 75cm (2ft 6in) of space between the upper and lower bunk. There should be a minimum clearance of 10cm (4in) between the upper surface of the mattress and the top of the guard rails. Finally, remind your children from time to time that bunk-beds are beds — not climbing frames or tree houses.

Upstairs windows are a particular danger for children. They should not be climbable or have a ledge large enough to sit on.

Furniture should never be left close to a window, which could allow children to reach the latch and open it. When windows are within children's reach they should be fitted with an automatic device to prevent them opening more than 10cm (4in). These devices should be designed so that they can be easily undone by an adult to provide the means of escape in the event of a fire. It is better to have windows that open higher up so that such devices are unnecessary. Discourage children from leaping or running close to windows. Accidents involving glass can lead to bad cuts, especially to the hands, wrists and face. Children have been killed from jagged glass penetrating the internal organs.

Toy safety

Injuries from accidents involving toys can be grouped under four categories: choking; cuts/bruises/fractures; poisoning; and burns. Most fatalities are caused by choking. The most common injuries are cuts and bruises or fractures arising from falls off toys such as rocking horses or bikes or from slipping on toys left lying around. Parents should look at the label before buying a toy. Don't ignore age warnings on the label. Small children and small parts don't mix. Keep older children's toys away from younger children. Educational toys such as chemistry sets may contain chemicals that are toxic or involve high temperatures. Throw broken toys away. Explain to children how to use their toys correctly and safely.

ROAD SAFETY

In 1991 twenty-three child pedestrians aged fourteen or younger were killed in road traffic accidents in Ireland, while the Garda Síochána recorded another 425 injured. Nine of the children killed were five years of age or younger. Ten children were killed on bicycles and eight were killed in cars.

Adults must remember that as a rule of thumb children are not developmentally ready to walk alone in areas where there is traffic until they are nine years of age. As cyclists, children under thirteen years of age cannot be expected to respond safely to an emergency when negotiating traffic. Many studies have shown that parents tend to overestimate their children's ability to cope with traffic.

Don't allow your children to play in dangerous areas, such as roads in which there are parked cars, where they may not be seen running out. A car hitting a child at 40mph will almost certainly kill the child, whereas a car travelling at 20mph almost certainly will not. Try to increase accident prevention awareness in your area and lobby your local politicians. *Educate* them to see the need for such traffic-calming measures as 'road humps' on residential roads.

WHEN AN ACCIDENT HAPPENS

Head injuries

If a child has had a major fall, for example from a bedroom window, or has been thrown some distance when struck by a car, it is important to remember that the spine may have been injured. Do not lift or move the child until the ambulance arrives. The whole of the spine must be kept in a straight line. This is best done with the child lying on his back. Stay with the child until help arrives. In the case of an unconscious child it may be necessary to open the airway as the tongue can drop back and obstruct it. This is done by gently pulling the chin forward.

Lesser falls, for example where a child falls out of a high chair or from a top bunk, do not usually cause unconsciousness, but the child often goes very white and may vomit or his eyes may twitch briefly. Where there is no concern about a spinal injury, a child should be placed in the 'recovery position', horizontal and on his side, until fully alert. Children will often rest quietly for an hour or two after a minor head injury, after which they come back to normal. If there is any period of unconsciousness lasting more than several seconds after the impact, if there is increasing headache or any change in the child's behaviour or awareness of his surroundings, he should be seen immediately by a doctor.

Poisoning

If you find your child with an opened bottle of tablets, look to see how many tablets are missing. If you think he has taken some but you are not sure if they are dangerous, phone the Poisons Information Centre (see Useful Services, p29) or bring your child immediately to a hospital Accident and Emergency Department or to your doctor, whichever is quicker. Do remember to bring the container and any remaining tablets with you.

If your child has swallowed some dangerous household substance, give him a glass of water to drink and then go immediately to the hospital. Do remember to bring the container with you.

If your child has splashed something dangerous in his eye, wash it out immediately with lukewarm water. Lie the child down, open the eye with your fingers and pour the water either from a jug or a hand-held shower in the bath. Continue rinsing the eye for ten minutes and then bring your child to be checked by your doctor or the Accident and Emergency Department.

The choking child

A child's airway can become obstructed by hard or soft objects. Never allow your child to run and eat at the same time, and discourage boisterous behaviour during meal times. A choking child will suddenly start coughing or may lose his voice completely. If a child is able to cough, it means that there is only partial obstruction and you should just watch him carefully, as his own efforts are the best means of clearing the airway. Total loss of voice or of cough means a complete obstruction. Do not put your finger blindly in a child's mouth while trying to clear it. This will only drive the object further down and increase the obstruction.

If an infant is choking, he should be placed face downwards over your lap while you sit with his head at a slight downward angle and his tummy resting on your thigh or arm. Give four firm slaps with the flat of your hand between the two shoulder blades. If this does not succeed in clearing the airway, turn the child over and give four similar thrusts on the lower centre chest. Look in the mouth, and if you can see the object remove it. If not, attempt to ventilate with mouth-to-mouth breathing. With a young infant it is easier to put your mouth over both his mouth and nose and blow gently in. Repeat these steps — back blows, chest thrusts, looking for the object and attempting to ventilate. The emergency services should be alerted immediately by phoning 999.

With an older choking child you will see him put his hand to his neck if the airway is obstructed. If it is partially obstructed and he is still coughing, allow him to clear the airway himself. If the airway is fully obstructed and the child is voiceless and cannot cough you should do the Heimlich Manoeuvre: stand behind him, make a fist with one hand, and with the thumb of this hand midway between the belly button and the rib cage in the midline of the body, grasp this hand with your other hand, encircling the child, and give four firm upward sharp thrusts. This may expel the object back up into the mouth. Look, and if you can see the object remove it. Do not search the mouth blindly with your finger. Attempt to ventilate using mouth-to-mouth breathing. If the child becomes unconscious, lie him flat on his back, kneel in the straddling position and repeat the abdominal thrust with the heel of your hand, upward in sharp jerks above the belly button. Repeat this sequence of thrusts, looking for the object and attempting to ventilate, until the ambulance arrives.

Broken bones

A child with a broken bone will be in a lot of pain, so do not move the limb unnecessarily. If it is an arm that is injured put it in a sling or support. If it is a leg, you can splint it by putting a little padding between his legs and tying the legs together before you move the child. Immobilisation requires that the joint above and below the injured area is splinted so that movement is not possible. If you have some pain-relieving medicine at home, give it to the child before you go to the hospital, particularly if you have some distance to travel.

Burns

If a child's clothing catches fire the Golden Rule is STOP, DROP and ROLL. Make the child lie down on the floor to stop the flames reaching his face, cover him with a rug or blanket to smother the flames, or roll him on the floor.

Scalds

Immediately, put the scald under cold running water, even before taking off the clothes. Once the water is running, take the clothes off and continue cold-water application for at least ten minutes. Cover the injury with a clean cotton cloth or kitchen 'cling film' — this reduces both the pain and the risk of infection. Call an ambulance or take the child to hospital, unless the burn is very minor. Never rub cream or ointment on a burn that needs medical attention, and don't prick the blisters.

Bleeding and bruises

If bleeding is severe, apply firm pressure on the bleeding area with your hand. Keep up the pressure for five minutes before checking if bleeding has stopped.

If a child has a nose-bleed, sit him upright and pinch the nose firmly high up, just where you can feel bone. Do not release the grip for ten minutes — watch the clock.

For smaller wounds, wash with antiseptic liquid. Make sure any grit or dirt is removed, then cover with a clean dressing. Go to your doctor or to the hospital if the wound is particularly deep or dirty, and you think stitches, further cleaning or a tetanus injection are needed.

For bruises or sprains apply a cold pack, for example a packet of frozen peas, and hold for ten minutes.

FIRST-AID KIT

Every household should have a first-aid kit, containing:

A box of *sticking plasters* in assorted sizes, eg Band-Aid

A small *bottle of antiseptic liquid,* eg Savlon or Dettol, which can be used to wash wounds.

Cotton wool — use with the antiseptic liquid to clean wounds.

A tube of *antiseptic cream,* eg chlorhexidine (Acriflex), to put on scrapes and cuts after cleaning.

Crepe bandages, 5cm and 7.5cm wide (2in and 3in) to be used to support sprained limbs.

Gauze squares, 10cm x 10cm (4in x 4in) — a small packet, to be put on cuts when cleaned.

Conforming bandages — 5cm and 7.5cm (2in and 3in), eg Mollelast, to wrap around the gauze square and keep bandage in place.

A large *triangular bandage,* to act as a sling.

Gloves — latex, available from chemists.

Scissors.

A safety pin.

Always keep paracetamol (eg Paralink, Calpol) and a thermometer in your home.

Useful services

Emergency — Fire, Garda, Ambulance: dial 999 (free of charge)
Poison Information Service, Beaumont Hospital, Dublin 9.
Tel. (01) 8379964/8379966

———————————

Dr Roisín Healy MRCP (Paed), FRCSI is Consultant in Accident and Emergency Medicine at Our Lady's Hospital for Sick Children, Crumlin, Dublin.

ANOREXIA AND BULIMIA

DR ANNE LEADER

In today's western world, fat is decidedly unfashionable. Fat people are often seen as ugly, lazy, stupid, greedy and undisciplined. On the other hand, thinness is equated with success, control, attractiveness and many other positive and alluring qualities.

As the so-called 'super models' get skinnier and more waif-like, increasing pressure is put on young girls to be as slim as possible. The huge effort required to achieve extreme thinness can lead to anorexia and bulimia. While boys occasionally suffer from these conditions, teenage girls are particularly at risk. Dr Anne Leader is a consultant psychiatrist, and an expert in eating disorders.

There is enormous prejudice against overweight people, particularly women. Several studies show that fat people are discriminated against in all areas of their lives and that being overweight is a serious social disadvantage. The famous quote 'You can never be too rich or too thin' sums up the present-day importance of slimness. Is it any wonder then that overweight women go to extreme lengths to avoid social disapproval? Anorexia and bulimia can be understood as desperate attempts to avoid obesity. Hilde Brüch — an authority on anorexia — captured the essence of the disease when she described it as a 'relentless pursuit of thinness'.

ANOREXIA NERVOSA

'Anorexia' is simply a medical term meaning 'loss of appetite'. Anorexia commonly occurs in a wide range of conditions, and is often one of the first signs of physical or mental illness. Anorexia nervosa, however, refers to a specific psychological condition with very definite signs and symptoms. The most important of these symptoms are weight loss, body image distortion, fat phobia, the loss of monthly periods (amenorrhoea), and an obsessive preoccupation with weight and shape.

Weight loss

The most striking outward sign of anorexia nervosa is dramatic weight loss. This is achieved by dieting, excessive exercising, vomiting, and in some cases over-use and abuse of laxatives and slimming tablets. Initially the diet is a straightforward weight-reducing diet, with the exclusion of 'fattening' foods. However, as weight is lost the diet becomes more extreme. Normal dieters are satisfied when they achieve their target. They have no desire to keep losing weight. Anorectics, on the other hand, cannot stop dieting, even when their original goals have long since been reached. They cannot 'let go' of the diet and it becomes an addiction over which they have no control. The more weight loss an anorectic achieves, the more she craves to be just a little thinner. Her desire for thinness is insatiable. As the disease progresses the diet becomes even more restrictive. Eventually she permits herself only tiny amounts of certain low-calorie foods. If she deviates from this regime, she is overwhelmed with guilt.

Over-exercising is another important method of achieving rapid weight loss. It is not unusual for anorectics to walk up to ten miles a day and engage in punishing workouts in the gym. The amount of energy these girls can have is quite remarkable. Even when cold, tired and hungry, anorectics feel compelled to carry out fanatical exercise routines. This compulsive exercising is not enjoyable, but is merely another task that must be completed in the ongoing quest for thinness.

The anorectic girl will try to hide the fact that she is eating so little. She will make excuses not to eat with the rest of her family, or with her friends. On the occasions when she cannot avoid family meals, she will probably say she is not hungry, busy herself serving others, take a small quantity of low-calorie food, and play around with the food rather than eat normally. This may lead to tension and arguments with her parents.

Vomiting occurs regularly in anorexia nervosa. It is commoner in anorectics who have a tendency to binge-eat on occasions. Anorectics construct their own perverse code of law when it comes to dieting. Certain foods are banned or 'illegal'. An enormous amount of mental energy is necessary to supervise these restrictions. From time to time most anorectics 'weaken' and consume 'forbidden' foods or eat more than the pre-ordained amount. Making themselves vomit is a way of ensuring that this increase in calories does not translate into weight gain.

The abuse of laxatives is also common in anorexia. Laxatives cause diarrhoea and weight loss. Taking large amounts of laxatives becomes a tempting solution for those who feel they have overeaten. Teenagers should never need laxatives, so parents should be concerned if they find empty packets of tablets in their bedroom.

Slimming tablets can also be abused, and doctors should always be very cautious about prescribing them.

Body image distortion

The second important symptom of anorexia nervosa is the inability to perceive the body as it really is. The full-blown anorectic sees herself as fat, despite being pathetically thin. In fact the thinner she becomes, the fatter she thinks she is. This is one of the central paradoxes of anorexia, and is called 'body image distortion'. It is an intrinsic part of the illness and no amount of arguing will have any effect on it. This is the one symptom that family and friends find most difficult to comprehend. In vain they try to convince the anorectic that she is seriously underweight. They cannot understand how she can still view herself as fat despite her obvious emaciation.

Because of 'body image distortion' the anorectic cannot believe she is thin. When she looks in the mirror she perceives a grossly distorted image of herself. This is a personal thing, and doesn't apply to other people — she sees them just as they are.

Fat phobia

Fat phobia is yet another symptom of anorexia. A phobia means an 'irrational fear'. Anorectics have a terror not only of becoming fat but of being a normal healthy weight. This fear of normal weight becomes understandable when body image distortion is taken into account. Ninety per cent of women are unhappy with their weight and shape, and fear fatness. The fat phobia that occurs in anorexia is a gross exaggeration of this fear.

Amenorrhoea

Loss of monthly periods (amenorrhoea) always occurs in anorexia nervosa. This is largely due to weight loss, but psychological factors may also play a part. The amenorrhoea happens when the anorectic loses more than 15 per cent of ideal body weight, when body fat content falls below some critical level for that individual.

Preoccupation with weight and shape

Anorectics enjoy no mental rest because any appetite that is denied tends to become more insistent. Although the word anorexia means 'loss of appetite', most anorectics in fact have a voracious appetite — so voracious that the power of their hunger terrifies them. Every waking moment must be given over to the control of that hunger. It must be dampened down, blocked out, controlled by will alone.

Anorectics have to be preoccupied with food at all times to guard against giving into temptation. They have a love-hate relationship with food. They long to be surrounded by it and delight in its sight and smell. Anorectics are often very competent cooks and have an encyclopaedic knowledge of calories. They love 'fattening up' family and friends while abstaining themselves. This iron discipline makes them feel morally superior to those lesser mortals who happen to enjoy their food! Eventually this preoccupation with food becomes overwhelming and dominates all mental activity. Anorectics complain that this obsessive thinking is one of the most disabling and depressing features of the illness.

BULIMIA NERVOSA

Bulimia nervosa is now the number one eating disorder. It is common in women in their twenties and thirties, but it also occurs in young girls. Anorexia nervosa is a very visible condition, whereas bulimia is a master of disguise. It is possible to hide bulimic symptoms from family and friends for several years.

The typical bulimic is a tense young woman who has been struggling unsuccessfully with weight for several years. Each time she diets she goes to more extreme lengths. Strict dieting leads to compulsive overeating. This type of yo-yo dieting is often the precursor of bulimia.

Binge-eating

The main symptom of bulimia is binge-eating. The main difference between binge-eating and comfort overeating is that the binger keeps on eating, even when it is no longer pleasurable. It has a compulsive quality and the binger feels that it is out of her control. Binges are followed by vomiting, laxative abuse, or periods of starvation. Like the anorectic, the bulimic has an abnormal relationship with food and has an obsessive interest in her appearance. Although it may fluctuate, the bulimic's weight, unlike the anorectic's, is usually within the normal range.

Compulsive eating often starts off as something that is done occasionally to alleviate stress and as a relief from strict dieting. Gradually bingeing becomes more frequent, and eventually takes place not only after meals but instead of them.

Compulsive eating is an interesting phenomenon and it is important to understand why people do it and why it is addictive. Food is a wonderful tranquilliser, and bingeing guarantees large quantities at frequent intervals.

Serotonin is an important brain chemical that is thought to be involved in controlling mood. There is evidence that carbohydrate deprivation decreases brain-serotonin levels. Low brain-serotonin levels are associated with anxiety states. Prior to the binge, the sufferer feels increasingly restless, agitated and out of control. These feelings are intensified if she has been dieting, which is often the case. One bulimic describes herself as resembling a 'cat on a hot tin roof' just prior to the binge. The compulsion to eat becomes unbearable, and in some cases the longer the binge is postponed the more excessive the final binge becomes.

The binge itself is initially intensely pleasurable and exciting. As eating progresses, the person feels more relaxed and settled. However, guilt feelings then begin to set in, and eating continues not for any additional relaxation but as a form of punishment. The binge experience is thus complex and varied. At first it is thrilling, then it is relaxing, and finally it is humiliating.

The experience of bingeing is also very liberating for some people. The dieter escapes not only from her dietary prison, but symbolically from all the petty frustrations and tyrannies of normal life. Many of these are real, but many are self-imposed due to her perfectionistic and rigid personality.

Bingeing is also a way of releasing pent-up aggressive feelings, which the bulimic is too polite to acknowledge in other ways. The language of bingeing is full of savagery and anger. Bulimics describe wolfing down food, devouring chocolates, etc. Bingeing itself is a frenzied and undignified behaviour and those who do it are ashamed of discussing its raw and animalistic nature.

When bingeing becomes a frequent occurrence, it is easy to understand how full-blown bulimia develops. A terrified girl who cannot contain her compulsive eating and who cannot condone the inevitable weight gain faces a dreadful dilemma. Vomiting seems to offer a seductive solution. Now the bulimic can continue to binge and at the same time preserve her treasured thinness. She can indulge and not bulge! She may start vomiting several times a day.

Vomiting, laxative abuse, obsessive exercise and periods of starvation all serve to control weight gain and soon become as addictive and necessary as the binge itself. Sometimes the person becomes excessively thin or even anorectic. On other occasions weight gain is excessive, and overweight becomes obvious.

As bulimia deepens, life revolves more and more around the addiction. The bulimic's mood is governed by the scales. When 'in control' of her eating, she feels powerful and successful. When bingeing, she is moody and depressed. Eventually she is completely ensnared by the bulimic bogey and, as one unfortunate victim so aptly described her plight, she cannot 'get out of the grip of the grub'.

Girls who develop bulimia become increasingly withdrawn from their family and friends. They have a horrible secret to hide, they may be spending long periods in the bathroom vomiting, and they may start stealing food from home. They may also begin to steal money from their parents to feed their addiction.

WHAT CAUSES EATING DISORDERS?

We do not know for certain what causes eating disorders. However, the overwhelming medical opinion supports the view that these illnesses are triggered by psychological factors. At a simple level they could be seen as extreme measures to prevent weight gain in young people with real or imagined weight problems. However, the situation is certainly more complex than this. There is an increased incidence of eating disorders, alcoholism, depressive illness and anxiety states in the families of those who suffer from eating disorders. This suggests that sufferers may have a genetic vulnerability to addictive conditions and neurotic illness.

We know that certain groups of people and certain personalities are more at risk. The majority of sufferers are young women. The seeds of the disease may be present from as early on as puberty. This is a time when girls put on extra weight and sexual development takes place. Anorexia in particular is often seen as a fear of sexuality and a general fear of growing up. Girls who are insecure about their bodies and who have low self-esteem often start dieting at this early age.

Exam pressures have never been greater. Anorectics in particular put huge pressure on themselves to succeed academically. When they fail to achieve unrealistic targets, they become unduly stressed. The year before the Leaving Certificate is definitely a time when young girls are prone to develop eating disorders.

Over-strict dieting is another risk factor in the development of eating disorders. It can lead to a pattern of eating very little. If the dieter breaks the strict diet, she may go on a binge for consolation, and this may be followed by self-induced vomiting.

MEDICAL COMPLICATIONS OF EATING DISORDERS

The main medical risk from anorexia nervosa comes from the effects of starvation on the heart and kidneys. The pulse rate is reduced due to an energy-conserving slowing of the metabolic rate. Blood pressure is also reduced, causing dizziness.

Vomiting, laxative abuse and the abuse of diuretics (drugs that trigger an increased production of urine) can cause sudden dramatic alterations in blood chemistry. These changes can in turn alter the rhythm of the heart. Sudden death may occur as a result of these 'arrhythmias'.

Vomiting also causes erosion of tooth enamel. In bulimia there is enlargement of the salivary glands in the face, giving a bloated appearance.

Bone loss is common in anorexia. This is known as osteoporosis — the same condition that affects women after the menopause. Fragile bones are more likely to break. If the illness occurs at an early age, the girl's bones may not grow fully and she may never reach her potential height.

In anorexia the skin is dry and scaly, and soft downy hair (lanugo hair) covers the arms, legs, back and face.

Chronic constipation is common in eating disorders, and the repeated use of laxatives may give rise to 'lazy' bowel.

The loss of monthly periods always occurs in anorexia.

It is important that all patients with eating disorders should have a full medical examination and an analysis of their blood chemistry.

TREATMENT

Weight management and stress management are the two cornerstones of successful treatment. The earlier the treatment is started, the better the outcome. Specialists who treat eating disorders only see the extreme cases. The majority of those who suffer from these conditions have mild or moderate forms, which can be dealt with by the patient's GP and the support of her family. It is very easy for a teenager with an eating disorder to become the focus of a huge family crisis. Parents naturally become very anxious when they realise that their daughter has this problem, but no amount of scolding, criticising or pressurising the girl to eat will solve the problem. Parents should try to adopt a calm, rational approach, despite their anxieties.

Weight management of anorexia

The first aim of treatment is to encourage weight gain. The anorectic's greatest fear is that if she starts to eat she will never stop. She has lost all confidence in her ability to commence eating and still control her appetite. For this reason she feels safer following a prescribed diet dictated by someone she can trust. A diet is constructed that will put on weight at roughly 1kg (2lb) per week. She is encouraged to eat three or four meals a day and to have a balanced, nourishing diet. Exercise is reduced to the minimum. She is reassured that if weight is put on slowly and safely she is much less likely to develop bulimia and overweight. She will also be encouraged to find that as weight goes on, body image distortion lessens and her obsession with food decreases.

Weight management of bulimia

The first aim of treatment in bulimia is to reduce the frequency and intensity of bingeing. If the bulimic keeps a food diary she can learn to identify the times and circumstances that cause her to binge. This can help her to avoid the triggers. When bingeing is down to three or four times a week or less, she should be actively encouraged to break the binge–vomit cycle.

It is almost impossible to give up vomiting and not expect to put on some weight. The bulimic must learn to accept weight gain as a temporary measure until she succeeds in controlling the bingeing. She should eat three or four regular nutritious meals each day, regardless of the intervening binges. Regular exercise prevents significant weight gain when vomiting has stopped.

Stress management

By and large people with eating disorders have high stress levels. Psychotherapy or 'talking therapy' can be very useful in alleviating stress. When problems are openly discussed, new solutions can be found. Sufferers can learn to recognise that their eating disorder is often a way of distracting themselves from other worries. If these worries can be solved, they may not need to comfort themselves with food (bingeing) or to switch off their worries with starvation (anorexia). Psychotherapy helps people develop a greater understanding and tolerance of themselves. Family therapy may also help.

Anorectics and bulimics find it very difficult to relax and need active encouragement to do so. They need to be given permission to let go of unnecessary commitments and to take 'time out' to develop leisure pursuits.

Women with eating disorders have a very negative and critical view of themselves. Recent research shows that they experience a slightly higher incidence of sexual abuse, which might explain their deep loathing of their bodies. Massage can be particularly helpful. Not only is it wonderfully relaxing, but it gives them a positive and pleasurable experience of their bodies.

Teenage girls should be encouraged to value the benefit of relaxation in the maintenance of good mental health. They should make out a list of all the activities they find enjoyable (other than eating), and should then be encouraged to 'binge' on these activities when they feel stressed, instead of turning to food.

Hospitalisation

In some cases, particularly in anorexia, the girl cannot get going on her own. She needs, for a time, the structure and support of hospital. This is particularly true if she is very underweight, is vomiting regularly or abusing large quantities of laxatives. It is also necessary if she is seriously depressed.

The putting on of weight is an essential element in the treatment of anorexia, and this is usually much easier in hospital. Bulimics also occasionally need hospitalisation, usually for shorter periods. An in-patient stay stabilises a chaotic eating pattern and nearly always succeeds in stopping bingeing and vomiting, at least temporarily.

Drugs can be very useful in the treatment of eating disorders as part of an overall treatment programme. The most commonly used drugs are antidepressants, which act by lowering anxiety levels.

They also lift the mood and lessen the compulsive force of bingeing or starvation.

A new group of antidepressants called the SSRIs (selective serotonin re-uptake inhibitors) has recently become available. These drugs have few serious side effects, and are not addictive. They are an exciting development in the treatment of eating disorders.

SELF-HELP GROUPS

Overeaters Anonymous is a self-help group for people who recognise the addictive nature of their eating habits. It is run roughly on the lines of Alcoholics Anonymous, and members follow a structured 'ten step' programme. Many people find regular OA attendance a highly valuable and necessary support in coping with their eating disorder.

PREVENTION

The best way to prevent eating disorders is to instil in our children a positive view of their bodies from an early age and enhance their confidence and self-esteem.

We can all control the local culture in our home, even if we cannot alter society as a whole. Comments about children's appearance should always be complimentary, regardless of their weight. Mothers who are themselves struggling with weight may be overly concerned about achieving thinness and perfection in their children. They must guard against contaminating their daughters with their own weight prejudice.

Food should be a neutral topic and should not be used to manipulate the behaviour of young children. When they require comfort or reward, non-food treats should be used as often as possible. In this way we can prevent programming children to turn to food when distressed. We should keep this in mind from the earliest age, for instance, try not to offer toddlers sweets to stop them crying. Instead of bribing kids with junk food, we should allow them to stay up late or watch a suitable video.

Meals should be regular, nutritious and pleasant. There should be no shortage of healthy food in the home. If children dislike certain foods, don't force them to eat these.

The enjoyment of exercise should be encouraged from an early age. Fat children avoid exercise for two reasons: they do not as a rule excel at sport; and exercise often involves exposure of the body, which makes them vulnerable to teasing. These children in particular should be helped to find a sport they are good at and can enjoy.

Teachers in secondary schools should have a high degree of awareness of the signs and symptoms of eating disorders. The dangers of strict dieting should be discussed in school and those who want to lose weight should be instructed on how to do so safely.

Parents should be sensitive and aware of any stresses their children are experiencing and discuss problems openly and frankly.

If there are signs of an eating disorder developing, it is best to seek help sooner rather than later. The dangers of vomiting and laxative abuse as a way of controlling weight must be explained. Compulsive eaters must be strongly warned not to go down this route.

Doctors, dietitians and counsellors all have a role to play in the treatment of eating disorders.

SIGNS AND SYMPTOMS OF EATING DISORDERS

Parents should suspect an eating disorder if they notice some of the following signs in their daughter (or son).

- She avoids eating with the family, yet she is very interested in cooking or baking.

- She continues on a strict diet after she has become thin.

- She starts wearing shapeless clothes to hide her figure, and avoids changing in front of others.

- She exercises obsessively.
- Her periods stop.
- As she gets very thin, downy hair appears on her face, arms, legs and back, and she feels the cold constantly.
- She vomits frequently.
- She takes laxatives and/or slimming tablets.
- There is evidence of bingeing — food missing from the kitchen, or empty packets of biscuits, chocolates, etc in her bedroom.
- She is depressed, withdrawn and has difficulty concentrating.

Useful address

Overeaters Anonymous, PO Box 2529, Dublin 5. Tel. (01) 4515138 (answering service for contact numbers nationwide)

Dr Anne Leader LRCSI, LRCPI, MRC Psych is a Consultant Psychiatrist attached to the Bons Secours Hospital, Glasnevin, Dublin. She specialises in the treatment of obesity and eating disorders.

BIRTH TO SIX WEEKS

DR WINIFRED A GORMAN

Bringing a new baby home is one of the most exciting events in life. But it can also be a terrifying experience, and can cause enormous anxiety for both experienced and first-time parents when they realise that they are now totally responsible for such a tiny creature.

Consultant paediatrician Dr Winifred Gorman highlights some of the problems and queries that may arise during the first six weeks of a child's life, and focuses in particular on those that may occur after discharge from the maternity unit.

The topics are presented in alphabetical order.

Bowel movements

Breastfed infants have a bowel movement after most feeds in the first one to two weeks, and after that the bowel movements become less frequent, but there are usually two to three per day. They are normally yellow in colour and soft.

Bottlefed infants have fewer bowel movements, which are harder and vary in colour from yellow to green to brown. (See also 'Constipation' and 'Diarrhoea'.) Frequency of bowel movements varies from two to three per day to one every two to three days.

Breastfeeding techniques

Breast milk is the most suitable food for the infant during the first six weeks of life. A healthy infant can be fed exclusively with breast milk for three to four months, without any vitamin supplements.

Getting breastfeeding established, especially for the first time, will require some help and support. Don't be afraid to ask the midwives in the hospital to help you, and when you return home, the advice and support of a friend who has successfully breastfed her baby will be invaluable. The La Leche League, a voluntary organisation dedicated to helping breastfeeding mothers, holds regular meetings nationwide (for address, see p120).

Before you begin breastfeeding, you should be in a comfortable position, either sitting comfortably in a chair or lying in bed. The baby should then be made comfortable, with his mouth facing the breast and at the same level as the breast. When you are in a sitting position, the baby's head, neck and back should be almost in a straight line. It may be necessary to put the baby on a cushion or pillow on your lap.

The infant should be allowed to find the nipple, and not have his cheeks pushed towards it. Babies have a rooting reflex, so that they will turn toward the side from which the stimulus comes. Gently take the nipple and stroke it across the infant's lips, and he will begin to root towards it. For effective nursing, the infant must get his lips over the areola (the pink or brown circle around the nipple). At first the baby may appear frantic, and seem unable to find the areola. Talking to him during these moments will help to calm him. By compressing the nipple and areola between the index and middle fingers, the breast can be made narrower so that the infant can place his lips around the areola. Make sure his nose is not compressed by the breast. The newborn infant breathes only through the nose, and may begin to cry or struggle because he can't breathe.

During and after feeding, massage around the entire periphery of the breast to prevent caking of the milk in the glands, which can lead to mastitis (inflammation of the breast) or 'breast abscess'. Caking usually occurs in the part of the breast nearest the armpit and feels like rocks or islands within the breast tissue. Massaging also helps to ensure that the infant gets the best quality milk.

Incomplete emptying of the breast also leads to mastitis, so it is important to change breasts regularly during feeding in order to ensure that both are emptied.

At the end of the nursing period, place a finger just inside the corner of the infant's mouth to break the suction, rather than pulling the nipple out of the baby's mouth, which may injure the nipple.

If the baby is premature or cannot be fed by the breast for a period of time, it is possible to express milk with the help of a breast-pump, and to freeze and store this until the baby is ready to use it. The midwives in the maternity hospital will show you how to express and store breast milk. The most effective breast-pumps are electric. They are available for rental at a fairly low cost. The Special Care Baby Units in the maternity hospitals can provide you with the names of the rental companies.

(See chapter on 'Feeding Your Child' for further information on breastfeeding.)

Circumcision

Some parents may choose circumcision for their son for religious or cultural reasons. Circumcision for medical reasons is almost never required in the first months of life. It is normal for the penis and foreskin to be fused at birth, and gradually become separate during the first few years of life. No attempt should be made to forcefully retract the foreskin or to clean underneath it. If the baby is passing urine normally, then there is no need for concern.

Colic

Colic is defined as bouts of irritability, fussing or crying, lasting for a total of more than three hours a day and occurring on more than three days in any week. Over 10 per cent of infants are colicky. Typically, the colicky infant is a fine healthy baby and a hungry feeder, but during or after feeds he develops a fit of crying and draws up his legs to his abdomen. The cause is unknown. The colic is usually at its worst in the evening time. Colic itself is completely harmless and almost always disappears by the age of four months.

Colic can be extremely difficult for tired and anxious parents to tolerate. Before deciding that your child has colic, ask your doctor to examine him to make sure there is nothing else making him cry. Once you are happy that the crying is a result of colic, then simply soothing the infant, walking with him over your shoulder, talking gently to him, are the types of measures to be adopted. Anti-colic drops, available from your pharmacy, can sometimes help.

Congenital hip dislocation

About fifteen per thousand infants will have this condition. The majority of loose or unstable hips will be diagnosed within the first few days of life, when the doctor does the baby's routine examination. Some, however, may later dislocate and may be diagnosed at later check-ups. The hip joint is unstable because the stabilising ligaments are lax. Treatment consists of simply stabilising the hip with a cloth pelvic harness until the joint itself becomes more stable. Babies who are in the breech position at term are more likely to have hip dislocation, and girls are four times more likely to be affected. Most unstable hips are perfect by three to four months old.

Constipation

Many healthy infants make lots of grunting noises and become very red in the face before they have a bowel movement. This is normal and does not mean that the baby is constipated. If the bowel movements are less frequent than every two days, or they appear very hard, then the baby can be given 55–85ml (2–3oz) of boiled water, with one to two teaspoons of sugar or glucose added. A little fresh orange juice added to this mixture may also help. The baby who is very constipated, with very hard bowel movements, may occasionally have a small amount of blood in the stools, resulting from a small tear in the anus (back passage). If this occurs, put plenty of Vaseline around the baby's back passage and this will protect it while it heals.

Cradle cap

This is a yellow scaly rash on the scalp, which sometimes spreads to the forehead, especially around the eyebrows, behind the ears, and the neck. It results from persistent oily secretions from the skin, and usually disappears by three months of age. It is never itchy and is not related in any way to eczema. It can be kept under control by using plenty of oil or aqueous cream on the scalp. This can be gently massaged into the scalp, then washed off after several hours. Frequent shampooing of the scalp with a baby shampoo or a special shampoo for cradle cap, available from your pharmacist, will also help.

Sometimes the rash spreads to the face and can look red and raised; usually a small amount of moisturising cream will keep this under control.

If cradle cap fails to clear or appears to be spreading, consult your doctor, as a prescription may be required.

Many infants have tiny yellow papules (pimples) over the nose, which disappear by about six weeks old. These also represent oily secretions from the skin, and if left alone will disappear completely.

Diarrhoea

Diarrhoea is uncommon in newborn babies and usually indicates an infection, such as gastro-enteritis. With diarrhoea, the bowel movements are watery in texture. Bowel movements that are green but not watery are completely normal and are not diarrhoea. Diarrhoea most commonly results from a viral infection, which can be highly contagious. It is particularly worrying if accompanied by vomiting, as the baby may rapidly become dehydrated (have insufficient body water). The risk of dehydration is higher in infants than in older children, and any infant under six weeks of age who develops diarrhoea should be seen promptly by a doctor. Your doctor will prescribe additional fluids for the baby — in the form of mineral-containing solutions, available from your pharmacist — or may admit the infant to hospital. (See also 'Nappy rash'.)

Eyes

A baby can see at birth, and will quite quickly start looking around with interest, especially at faces and coloured objects. The eyes may be puffy at birth, but this swelling disappears rapidly. Bruises in the whites of the eye (sclera) commonly occur as a result of delivery, are usually harmless and disappear within two to three weeks.

The eyes may be blue, green, grey, or brown at birth, but may change gradually. The permanent eye colour will be apparent by six months of age. If one or both pupils is grey or opaque, the baby may have a cataract, but this is very uncommon.

Newborn babies often have rather runny or sticky eyes. This results from a blocked tear duct, and frequently the eyes do not clear up fully until the child is five to six months old. In the meantime they should be cleaned regularly with clean cotton swabs dipped in cooled boiled water. It is important to clean each eye with a fresh swab. The eye itself should look clear and healthy, without any redness in the white of the eye.

If the eye becomes very pussy, with copious yellow to green secretions, medical attention should be sought, as the baby may have an eye infection. (See chapter on 'Eyes'.)

Feeding

Food is the most immediate and most basic need of the healthy newborn infant. An infant who is feeding well and is gaining weight steadily is unlikely to have a serious medical problem. (See chapter on 'Feeding Your Child' for information on breastfeeding and bottlefeeding. Also 'Breastfeeding techniques' above.)

Hernias

a) Umbilical hernia: it is common for young infants to have a protruding navel. Frequently there can be quite a large bulge, which becomes even larger when the baby cries. This is an umbilical hernia. It is completely harmless and will gradually become smaller and usually disappear. No treatment is necessary or desirable in infancy.

b) Groin (inguinal) hernia: if there is a swelling in the groin, then the baby may have an inguinal hernia. In a baby boy, the swelling develops in the groin and may spread downwards into the scrotum. It may at first be intermittent and only visible when the baby cries. An inguinal hernia is much less common in girls, but similarly the main symptom is a groin swelling. Any such swelling should be discussed with your doctor promptly. An inguinal hernia always requires surgical correction. The baby will be in hospital for one day, and will not normally need to stay overnight.

Jaundice

More than 50 per cent of newborn infants have some jaundice in the first week of life. Jaundice is a yellow discoloration of the skin that gives the newborn baby a healthy, 'tanned' appearance. It results from an accumulation of pigments in the skin due to a temporary immaturity of the baby's system after birth. Mild jaundice is completely normal in the vast majority of healthy infants, and many breastfed infants remain slightly jaundiced for two to three weeks.

Some newborn babies are more severely jaundiced. This mainly occurs where there is a difference between the blood groups of mother and infant. The baby may be treated in hospital by lying him under a light similar to sunlight for one to two days.

If jaundice continues for more than two weeks, and is accompanied by very pale bowel movements and/or very dark coloured urine, medical attention should be sought, as the baby may have a rare and possibly serious problem.

Nappy rash

Nearly every infant develops a nappy rash at some stage during the first six weeks of life. Contributory causes include wet nappies and warmth. The baby often has a yeast (thrush) infection, which aggravates the rash. Thrush infection will require a prescription medicine from your doctor.

Babies with diarrhoea may have nappy rash because of local irritation from the frequent bowel movements. The rash usually improves rapidly if the nappy is left off as often as possible to allow air to get to the skin. A protective barrier cream may also be helpful if the irritation is severe.

Rashes

Rashes often occur within the first six weeks of life, and most are harmless and soon disappear. The full-term newborn often has a blotchy red rash on his body, interspersed with small white pustules (pimples) in the first few days of life. This may look quite dramatic, but is completely harmless, and will normally have disappeared by the seventh day.

Minor rashes of red spots may occur on the face, front of the chest and neck during the first six weeks. These result from a combination of warm clothing and sweating, and are totally harmless.

Sleeping

During the first weeks of life, most infants will sleep from twelve to eighteen hours per day. There is no absolute minimum or maximum period that an infant needs to sleep for, but intervals of three to four hours sleep, with intervening episodes of wakefulness for one to two hours, could be considered typical in the newborn. Babies, however, rapidly become more alert as the weeks go by, and will very quickly learn to enjoy being picked up and given individual attention.

From two to three weeks of age onwards you should try to encourage the baby to sleep more during the night. Night-time wakefulness should be for feeding (and changing) only, after which the baby should be put back down. Picking the baby up again, even if he is crying, should be resisted as far as possible. As long as the baby is feeding adequately, which can be confirmed by weighing the baby (see 'Weight gain'), there is no reason why he should not be actively encouraged to sleep through the night by six weeks of age. Establishing a routine will help both the baby and the parents — the baby will generally be happier if the parents are less fatigued, and the parents' wellbeing is vital if they are to have the energy to care for the baby in a relaxed manner.

The baby should be put to sleep on his side. It can be helpful to place a rolled-up towel behind the baby's back to prevent him rolling over, but do remember to change it to the other side each time you put him down to sleep, so that he is not always sleeping on the one side.

Never use a pillow with a small baby. (See also chapter on 'Sleep Problems'.)

Snuffles

Most babies have stuffy noses from time to time. Breathing may be very noisy 'like a train', and may sound particularly alarming in the quiet of the night. The snuffles occur as a result of the baby's small nasal passages and his inability to clear the nose himself. If the baby is feeding well despite the snuffles, there is no need for concern. Sneezing, hiccups and yawning are common and normal occurrences in young babies.

Temperature and warmth

A room temperature that is comfortable for an adult in indoor clothing is suitable for a baby. Most babies will be very comfortable in a vest, all-in-one babysuit and several blankets. In summer, two to three blankets are usually adequate, whereas in winter some extra layers may be needed. It is not necessary or desirable to cover the baby's head or to wrap the baby tightly.

Normal body temperature is about 36.9°C (98.4°F). Babies' temperatures are often taken 'rectally' — that is, by inserting a clinical thermometer into the back passage and holding it there for a minute. This should be done with great care, and it is advisable to have a doctor show you how to do this.

If the baby feels unusually warm, check the rectal temperature. If the temperature is above 100°F or 37.5°C, make sure that the baby is not overwrapped. You should unwrap the baby, and if the temperature is still high after an hour, call your doctor or maternity hospital. A temperature in a baby less than six weeks old *always* requires medical attention.

Vomiting or regurgitating (possetting)

Some vomiting or regurgitation of food is a normal occurrence in the healthy infant. It frequently begins in the first week of life. Typically, the baby feeds well, but during or after the feed brings back a small amount. This usually occurs immediately after the feed, but it can happen up to several hours later. The vomiting is often, though not always, preceded by wind or colic. The vomit may appear much larger in volume than it actually is (try spilling one or two ounces of milk on an old cloth to give you an idea!).

The key points to check, with a baby who is vomiting or spitting up regularly, are that the baby is gaining weight and is having regular bowel movements and wet nappies. In a small minority of cases, vomiting may be a sign of a medical problem, such as pyloric stenosis. A pyloric stenosis is a thickening of the muscle at the exit from the stomach. This is not normally present at birth, but typically develops at two to three weeks of age. With a pyloric stenosis, the vomiting is often projectile, that is, the baby vomits suddenly and with such force that the vomited material ends up several feet away. It is more common in male infants and may require surgery. If there is a change in the baby's usual pattern of vomiting, or if a baby who has never or only rarely vomited, suddenly starts to vomit every feed, you should consult your doctor or maternity hospital.

Urinary tract infection

A baby who has a urinary tract infection may vomit. He will usually also be unwell, possibly with a temperature, and will be uninterested in his feeds. This condition is treated with antibiotics, by a doctor.

Weight gain

Most infants lose up to 10 per cent of their body weight within the first week of life. This is because at delivery the body contains extra water, which is eliminated during the first week. After that the baby should gain about 200g (7oz) per week, so that by six weeks of age he should be about 0.5kg to 1.5kg (1–3lb) above the birth weight. Some babies gain more, but this is rarely a cause for concern. Inadequate weight gain on the other hand, i.e. less than 0.5kg (1lb) in six weeks, should be investigated so that a cause can be identified.

WHEN TO CALL THE DOCTOR

If a small baby appears generally unwell, it is advisable to 'play safe' and call the doctor. Always call the doctor if the child shows the following symptoms:

- Refusal of more than one feed.

- Rectal temperature of more than $37.5^{\circ}C$ ($100^{\circ}F$).

- Vomiting that comes on suddenly and occurs with most feeds.

- No weight gain at two to three weeks old.

- Jaundice lasting more than two weeks, especially if bowel movements are very pale in colour.
- A swelling in the groin, suggesting a hernia.
- A grey, opaque pupil in either eye, suggesting a cataract.
- Sudden lethargy and disinterest in surroundings.
- Diarrhoea.
- Pussy discharge from eyes.

———————————————

Dr Winifred A Gorman BSc, DCH, FRCPI, FAAP is Consultant Paediatrician at the National Maternity Hospital, Holles Street, Dublin, and Our Lady's Hospital for Sick Children, Crumlin, Dublin.

BONES AND JOINTS

MR MICHAEL M STEPHENS

The types of problems that children can have in their bones and joints are very different from those that affect adults. While adults may suffer from conditions such as arthritis and slipped discs, childhood orthopaedic conditions include congenital hip dislocation, flat feet, scoliosis, knock-knees, etc. Orthopaedic surgeon Mr Michael Stephens describes these conditions and how they can be treated.

SPINAL PROBLEMS

Scoliosis

The normal spine is straight, having a slight hollow in the neck, a convexity or slight roundness in the chest, and a hollow in the small of the back. Scoliosis is a deformity in which the spine curves to one side or the other. It usually starts in childhood and is more common in girls. The cause is usually unknown.

Many children have minor curvature of the spine, which is not significant, but it is important to have this checked by a general practitioner. Screening programmes are now conducted in schools, where specially trained people examine children and, if necessary, refer them for further investigation.

Scoliosis is normally painless, and if pain is a feature, this must be discussed immediately with your doctor. A small percentage of children with scoliosis are at risk of developing a severe deformity, and will have to wear a brace for a short period of time. A proportion of these children will eventually require surgery. Surgery is often delayed until the skeleton is mature, which may be about fifteen years of age in a female and sixteen or seventeen in a male.

Other spinal conditions

Any abnormal skin pigmentation or a hairy patch in the low back area may indicate spinal abnormalities, and should be brought to the attention of your doctor.

A mild hump or roundness in the upper spine is usually caused by bad posture, but it can indicate abnormalities of growth in the vertebrae (bones that form the spine), so it is advisable to have it checked out by your doctor. In rare instances it may require bracing.

Back pain is rare in children and, if persistent, will require medical assessment. A slipped or prolapsed disc is unlikely to occur in a young child, but can occur occasionally in a teenager. When diagnosed it will usually be treated with bed-rest, pain-killers and special exercises. Surgery is rarely required.

DISORDERS OF THE UPPER LIMBS

Erb's palsy

It is unusual for a child to develop problems in the upper limbs, but occasionally at birth an arm may be weak. This condition is called Erb's palsy, and may be due to a difficult labour. It is often a major concern for parents, but the condition generally improves with time, although it can take over a year for the child to recover fully.

Shoulder click

Shoulder dislocation is rare in children, but some children can have the sensation of a 'click' in the shoulder, as if it is going in and out. This is due to general looseness of the joint, and is commonly called multi-directional instability. It does not require treatment, and often the shoulder becomes stable as the child nears full maturity at around fifteen or sixteen. It is important that a child with this sensation doesn't continually click the shoulder as a 'party piece', as this may prolong the symptoms and delay natural recovery.

Trigger-thumb

Trigger-thumb is a common disorder of the hand, seen in early childhood. This is where the thumb remains bent at the joint above the nail, and can't straighten fully. It happens because the tendon that bends the thumb gets caught in its tunnel at the base of the thumb. It is so-called because in the early stages it can click in and out as the child tries to bend and straighten the thumb. This condition is easily treated by surgical release of the tendon through a small incision at the base of the thumb — an operation that can generally be carried out in one day (see 'Day-care surgery', p82).

Extra or missing fingers

Children born with extra fingers may require surgical correction, and this is generally very successful. Some children are born missing a finger, and since they know nothing else, they usually manage very well. Occasionally, one of the fingers will have to be repositioned to improve the grip.

Upper limb deficiency

A very small number of children are born with part of a hand or arm missing. They may require surgery to improve the position of the arm or the grip, or a prosthesis (artificial arm or hand) either for cosmetic purposes or to assist them with everyday tasks.

DISORDERS OF THE LOWER LIMBS

Dislocation of the hips

Sometimes a paediatrician examining a newborn baby will feel the hip to be loose or unstable, and will hear a 'click' when the hip is moved. In the past this was given the name CDH (congenital dislocation of the hip). Generally it is not a true dislocation, but rather a looseness of the hip. Girls are affected four times as often as boys. The cause is unknown, but it happens more often in babies who have a breech birth, and it can run in families. If the condition is not detected and treated early, the child may develop a limp. To stabilise the limp, splints or a cloth pelvic harness may be used on the child for two to four months; the harness will hold the ball of the hip-joint in its socket so that it can develop properly. This treatment usually works, and the child is able to walk normally, with no after-effects. However, a certain number of hips develop with a poor socket, and slowly over the ensuing year the hip may dislocate. The commonest symptom of this type of problem is that the legs cannot be brought fully apart. Many of these hips correct themselves as the child gets older, but x-rays may be required to monitor the development. Occasionally some form of surgery is required to deepen the socket.

Perthes' disease

Perthes' disease is a condition that can affect the hip when the child is three to six years of age. The symptoms include pain and a limp.

For some unknown reason the blood supply to the hip becomes diminished, so that the ball of the hip joint becomes soft and flat. It occurs in boys more than girls, and usually only one hip is affected. Many children with this condition require observation only, because as the hip grows the problem rectifies itself. Surgery is required occasionally if the ball of the hip joint doesn't remain within the socket.

Slipped epiphysis

Between the ages of ten and sixteen, a condition called slipped epiphysis can affect the hip. This is where the growing part of the hip joint (the epiphysis) slips off the top shaft of the femur or thigh bone. It is more common in tall or overweight children, and may come on gradually, or quickly, usually spontaneously or after an injury. It is a serious condition that requires urgent treatment. It is complicated by the fact that in the early stages the child may not complain of pain around the hip, but may complain of pain in the knee. The diagnosis is made with an x-ray, and the treatment involves inserting a pin to prevent the epiphysis slipping any further. This is carried out under a general anaesthetic.

Knock-knees and bow-legs

Knock-knees and bow-legs are commonly seen in young children and babies, and must be classed as a normal variation rather than a true deformity. Although these conditions are often of major concern to parents, the vast majority of children grow out of them as the legs develop. It may, however, take many years for the legs to become what we adults regard as normal.

In-toeing

In-toeing, when the child walks with the feet turned in, is one of the commonest reasons for referral to an orthopaedic clinic. Generally the legs are of normal shape and there are no foot abnormalities. It can really be classified as a postural deformity, and it arises because the whole leg is turned in from the hip down. This happens because the hip joint is slightly rotated, which allows the legs to turn in. Some of these children can sit on the ground with their knees bent and the calf and feet completely turned out on each side; this has been described as the 'reversed tailor position'— the opposite to cross-legged. They should be discouraged from sitting in this position because it slows down the body's natural remodelling process, which will ultimately correct the problem without the necessity for further treatment. In the past, shoes with raised insteps were recommended, but research has shown this treatment to be of little value.

Talipes equinovarus (club-foot)

This is a birth defect in which the foot is turned in and down. It is the commonest serious condition affecting the foot. The term 'club-foot' is old-fashioned and derogatory, and should be discarded. There are various grades of the condition, from mild to severe, and it is twice as common in boys.

Initial treatment in the newborn is with manipulation of the foot and ankle, with splints, taping, and sometimes plaster. The minor forms are often completely corrected by such treatment. At the end of six weeks, the more severe forms will not be fully corrected, and further treatment will often be carried out over the ensuing months. This can sometimes involve minor surgical procedures, such as lengthening the heel cord, or more extensive procedures, such as releasing all the tight structures on the inner side of the foot. In many cases the more extensive treatment is delayed until about nine months of age. After the surgery a plaster is applied for a period of three months, and occasionally pins are inserted and left in the foot for the first six weeks following surgery. This means that the cast is removed when the child is about one year old, when walking will stimulate growth and movement within the foot. In the severe forms, further surgery may be required in later years. The aim of surgery is to alter the foot so that it will be flat on the ground when the child walks.

A child with talipes equinovarus may also have a thin calf, and this is more noticeable if the talipes deformity is on one side only.

The foot may also be smaller, and unfortunately surgery cannot correct either the size of the calf or the size of the foot.

Calcanius deformity

This is the opposite of talipes equinovarus; the child is born with the feet turned out, to an excessive degree. Unlike talipes equinovarus this is not a serious condition, and by the age of one year it is often significantly better, and has practically disappeared by the age of two. Occasionally, all it requires is gentle stretching in the early stages. A physiotherapist will instruct the parent on how to do this.

Flat feet

Flatfootedness is normal for a baby. As the child walks, gets stronger, and muscles develop, the arches form. This type of flatfootedness only needs attention if the feet are stiff. If the feet are still flat at the age of ten to twelve, they should be assessed. If they are flexible and not painful, they usually require no treatment; a certain percentage of the adult population has flat feet, with no accompanying problems. Arch supports in the shoes, and strengthening exercises, may help to make walking and standing more comfortable. Surgery is not usually required unless the feet are stiff and painful, which may indicate an abnormality in the bones of the feet.

Bone and joint infection

Infection in bones and joints is not an uncommon problem in childhood. Infection in bones is known as osteomyelitis, and in joints it is known as septic arthritis. Both cause a rise in temperature, pain and a limp. Infection usually affects the lower limbs, but can involve the upper limbs and, very occasionally, the spine (discitis). It requires intensive treatment with antibiotics at an early stage, usually in hospital.

Osteomyelitis is treated with intravenous antibiotics, and surgery is rarely required unless an abscess is present. The child is normally kept in hospital until the infection settles and blood tests return to normal. This may take from one to three weeks, and antibiotics are then continued orally for a total of six weeks.

With septic arthritis, the joint generally has to be surgically drained to clean out the pus. Once this is carried out, treatment is the same as that outlined for osteomyelitis. The infected limb is often splinted with plaster to allow it to heal.

FRACTURES

Children's bones react to trauma and fractures in a completely different way from the bones of adults. Since the fractures are occurring in bones that are growing, these bones have a great potential to remodel. For example, when a child breaks an arm, it often knits with a bend, but in a matter of three to nine months the bend will completely remodel, and an x-ray taken some years after will show no trace of the fracture.

Fractures in children are usually treated with plaster; screws and plates are rarely required. The period in plaster depends on the age of the child and the type of the fracture, but generally speaking the younger the child, the shorter the period. For example, a fractured wrist in a one-year-old may only require a plaster for one to two weeks, whereas in a ten-year-old it may be required for five weeks. Fractures of the femur or thigh bone pose a particular problem. Some can be put in plaster immediately while others may require hospitalisation and traction (the leg is stretched with a series of weights and pulleys) for a period of several weeks. Once the fracture has started to join, a plaster or splint is applied to allow the child to go home.

LIMPING

The development of a limp in childhood is a common problem and accounts for many of the attendances in accident and emergency departments. Apart from injury, limping may result from many of the conditions outlined above, for example, infection in bone and joints, Perthes' Disease, congenital dislocation of the hips, or slipped epiphysis. The most common cause is a condition known as irritable hip. This is usually diagnosed when other problems have been ruled out, and is generally characterised by irritation, inflammation or fluid around a hip. It normally gets better in time and may only require bed-rest, though sometimes traction will be required, and this may necessitate a stay in hospital.

Mr Michael Stephens, FRCSI, MSc (Bio Eng), is Consultant Orthopaedic Surgeon at The Children's Hospital, Temple Street, Dublin.

BREATHING PROBLEMS

PROFESSOR GERRY LOFTUS

Coughs and sneezes
Spread diseases,
Cover your mouth
By using your handkerchief

These were the words of advice on a public health poster that I remember from my childhood. Although public health warnings in the Nineties are much more likely to highlight the dangers of AIDS or passive smoking, coughs and sneezes still fill the air with germs, especially in winter. As Professor Gerry Loftus, consultant in paediatric respiratory medicine, explains, children can be affected by many different breathing problems.

BREATHING PROBLEMS

The newborn infant lives in a germ-free environment throughout pregnancy. Following delivery, the baby comes into contact with many germs. The antibody levels in the baby's blood at birth are the same as his mother's, and will protect him against most of the infections that the mother has had in her lifetime. This antibody protection lasts for three to six months. Thereafter, infants will have seventy to ninety significant respiratory infections in the course of childhood, almost all of them viral infections, such as colds, croup, etc. The frequency of infections peaks between the ages of five and seven years, after which it declines. These infections may be viewed as 'immune education' and are regarded as a normal part of childhood.

When infection invades the respiratory tract, illness may result. Germs inflict damage, and the body's defences fight back. The immune system, which is the body's defence system, recognises germs as enemies, and causes the lymph nodes (glands) to manufacture antibodies, which kill the germs and give future immunity against the infection. Lymph nodes enlarge when they are actively manufacturing, and these can often be felt in the neck — at the sides, just below the angle of the jaw. When the body has eliminated the germs the 'swollen glands' recede. Since infections occur frequently, the lymph tissues around the respiratory tract are kept busy. For this reason, enlargement of the tonsils, the adenoids, and the lymph nodes in the neck occurs often during childhood.

Infections are usually acquired from other children and their frequency will depend on the degree of exposure. For example, a child living alone with his parents in a remote area may have very few illnesses until he starts school, then he will have almost constant coughs and colds as a result of increased exposure and his 'poorly educated' immune system.

The vast majority of the normal infections of childhood are trivial, giving rise to few or no symptoms. Infections are more troublesome in children under one year, and in those whose health is already compromised by poor nutrition or living conditions.

Passive smoking, especially during pregnancy, increases the risk of serious respiratory illness in childhood. If the mother smokes during pregnancy, the developing infant's lungs are exposed to high levels of nicotine and carbon monoxide. These compounds appear to interfere with normal lung growth and development.

Breastfeeding gives protection against respiratory illness in early infancy, when the child is most vulnerable. Effective, safe immunisation can prevent serious illnesses such as whooping cough (pertussis), measles, and epiglottitis (HIB), and it is every parent's duty to ensure that children are fully immunised. (See chapter on 'Infectious Diseases'.)

Sneezes and sniffles

When we breathe, air enters through the nose and mouth, and passes through the throat, the windpipe and the breathing tubes in the lungs. These breathing tubes branch many times, ultimately leading to tiny air sacs, through which oxygen enters the blood and carbon dioxide leaves. The respiratory (breathing) passages may be divided into three parts: upper — nose and throat; middle — windpipe, which can be felt at the front of the neck; and lower — the branching tubes in the chest.

Abnormal breathing noises depend on where the infection is located — sneezes and sniffles indicate a problem in the upper airway, while coughs and wheezes are lower airway problems. Since germs, particularly viruses, do not observe strict demarcation, there is frequently overlap between upper, mid and lower respiratory problems.

A sneeze is a sudden expulsion of air which clears secretions from the upper airways. It is a defence mechanism aimed at eliminating an enemy, be it infection or irritation. Sneezes usually occur with upper respiratory infection or nasal allergy.

Sniffles are noisy nasal breath-sounds due to excessive secretion in the nose. This excessive secretion may be a normal feature in small infants, or result from infection (usually viral) or allergy.

Most 'colds' are viral infections of the upper airway. The child will usually have a slight fever, with sneezing, running nose and perhaps a slight cough. These viral infections are extremely common and are transmitted from person to person by droplets spread via coughs and sneezes, or by hand-to-hand contact. The advice 'never shake hands with a person who has a cold' is sound. Simple viral colds do not require any specific treatment, but if the child is uncomfortable, paracetamol and hot drinks are helpful.

Allergic rhinitis or hayfever may also give rise to sneezing and sniffles. Symptoms are usually present in the pollen season, but may occur all year round. Affected individuals will normally have a chronically blocked and dripping nose, and may have the appearance of black rims under their eyes — the so-called 'allergy shiners'. This condition may respond to antihistamines or preventive nasal sprays. Ask your family doctor about these treatments.

Stridor

This is a high-pitched noise made when the mid respiratory tract is narrowed. It sounds like the initial 'hee' of a donkey's 'hee-haw'. It is most prominent when breathing 'in'. Stridor may be due to a narrowing that is present from birth, or to infection or an inhaled foreign body, for example a coin or peanut.

In most cases a viral infection of the mid respiratory tract is responsible. These children also have a 'croupy' barking cough and are hoarse. This condition is usually not serious and recovers spontaneously. Parents are often advised to allow the 'croupy' child to inhale steam. This form of treatment is usually of little value, and may expose the child to the risk of burns from boiling water.

Epiglottitis

Epiglottitis is a rare, potentially fatal infection of the mid airway. The child becomes rapidly unwell, with stridor and a high fever. He will be unable to swallow, and be drooling saliva, gasping for air, with no cough, and a voice that is muffled rather than hoarse. These children require urgent referral to hospital. Fortunately this illness is now preventable with HiB immunisation. (See chapter on 'Infectious Diseases.')

Coughs

A cough is produced by forcefully breathing out against a partially closed airway. It produces a powerful expulsive movement of any mucus or foreign material in the breathing passages. The cough is a protective reflex and an important part of normal airway hygiene. It is brought on when cough receptors are stimulated by excessive mucus, infection, irritant smoke or particles. Sputum (phlegm or spit) is a mixture of germs and mucus that is cleared from the airway during infection. Most young children swallow sputum when it is coughed up. This is far more hygienic than the adult habit of spitting it up, but because it is swallowed it tends to accumulate in the stomach and may be vomited up later. Prolonged coughing often triggers vomiting in children.

Whooping cough (pertussis) produces particularly distressing spasms of coughing. With this illness the child appears to have a cold for three to four days, and then progresses to uncontrollable, prolonged spasms of coughing, going red or blue in the face, vomiting and whooping as he breathes in rapidly to inflate the lungs, which have been squeezed empty. The illness can cause severe spasms of coughing and vomiting for two to three weeks, and then an increased tendency to cough for several months afterwards. There is no effective treatment, but the condition is preventable with immunisation. (See chapter on 'Infectious Diseases'.)

A recurrent cough, particularly when it occurs at night, after exercise, or is accompanied by wheeze, is suggestive of asthma.

The treatment of a cough should be directed at the cause. Since the cough is a helpful protective mechanism, it is usually not advisable to suppress it. Coughs are mainly caused by viral infections. These are mild and usually short-lived. Viral infections require no specific treatment as they will get better themselves. When coughs are due to bacterial infections, they are normally accompanied by fever, loss of appetite and green phlegm, and an antibiotic is usually prescribed. Cough bottles do not influence the rate of recovery from the illness and appear to be no more effective in relieving symptoms than giving the child plenty of drinks.

Serious chest infection may be present with little or no cough. Children with lobar pneumonia, for example, usually develop an abrupt illness. They will have a high fever and be generally very unwell. They will often have chest pain, which worsens when they take a deep breath. Antibiotic treatment is necessary.

Wheezes

Wheeze is a musical noise produced by a turbulent flow of air in narrowed airways. The narrowing may be due to infection, an inhaled foreign body, or, most commonly of all, asthma. In infancy, approximately 20 per cent of babies will wheeze at some stage. This is mainly related to viral infection. Bronchiolitis is a wheeze-associated viral infection of the chest that occurs in epidemic proportions each winter. One to two per cent of all infants are hospitalised with this infection, and these babies may be prone to recurrent wheeze for several weeks or months afterwards. In general, however, wheeze disappears before the second birthday.

In later childhood, wheeze usually means asthma, particularly if the wheeze is recurrent, triggered by colds and exercise, and is worst at night. Some 10 to 15 per cent of children are affected by asthma. In most cases it is mild and episodic, and clears up completely before the teens. A minority of children have frequent attacks or persistent symptoms on a daily basis. Effective safe treatments are available, the type and combination depending on the severity of the illness. Certain medications will relieve the tightness, while others will prevent symptoms. Your doctor will be able to decide which treatment is most appropriate for your child. If the child is given an inhaler, then it is important that it be used properly.

Avoidance of passive smoking is important in controlling asthma. Though allergy has a role in the cause of childhood asthma (for example, some children are allergic to grass pollen or house mites), unless there is an obvious connection with a particular food, diets are of no value. Immunotherapy and desensitisation injections are generally viewed as dangerous and useless.

An inhaled foreign body is a rare but important cause of sudden-onset wheeze. Peanuts are a common culprit, and for this reason they should never be given to children under the age of seven.

WHEN TO CONSULT YOUR DOCTOR

- In infants, the following symptoms are suggestive of a serious illness: very high fever, excessive sleepiness, food and drink refusal, breathlessness, or an anxious, worried appearance.

- In older children, the presence of a high fever, chest pain, breathlessness and general upset would indicate the need to consult your doctor.

- Where the child has developed sudden-onset stridor without a cough and with salivary drooling, he should be taken to hospital immediately.

- Recurrent infections may be indicative of serious illness if they are accompanied by weight loss, diarrhoea or other infections.

- If the child's respiratory symptoms are causing frequent school absence and interfering with exercise and sleep, help should be sought.

- You should also consult your doctor if your child persistently produces green phlegm or has any abnormality in the shape of the chest.

P B G Loftus MD, FRCPI, DCH is Professor of Paediatrics at University College Hospital, Galway.

CHILDREN IN HOSPITAL

DR JOHN F A MURPHY

Children's hospitals today are bright, colourful places, with an air of cheerful chaos. There are lots of parents in the wards, there are toys scattered everywhere, and doctors and nurses often have to go looking for their patients when it is time for a treatment or examination.

But it wasn't always like this. Until the 1950s children's wards were organised like adult wards, with an emphasis on orderly routines and very strict visiting hours. Consultant paediatrician Dr John Murphy explains how these changes came about and how parents can make their children's stay in hospital as easy as possible.

THE CHILDREN'S HOSPITAL

The present enlightened approach towards the care of children in hospital took a long time to evolve. Children's hospitals were founded at the turn of the century in response to the needs of the large numbers of children suffering from infectious diseases and malnutrition.

In the early days, hospitals were places that children went in to and subsequently came back from; professionals revealed very little about hospital procedures; parents didn't know what was happening because they were not permitted to visit their children; and the children themselves were too young to relate their experiences and express their emotions. Hospitalisation often had a damaging effect, and after a stay in hospital many children suffered from nightmares, bedwetting, poor school performance, and clinging, insecure behaviour. These problems bore little relationship to the length of stay in hospital, and they could be profound after even a short admission. Initially these effects of hospitalisation were attributed to a variety of factors, but it was gradually realised that the main component was separation from parents. The historic British Platt Report on Hospitalisation Policy of 1959 noted the importance of visiting children in hospital and the provision of beds for mothers to stay with the younger children. It took a long time, however, before this was accepted by hospital authorities because they feared that the sheer numbers would interfere with the running of the ward.

A letter written to the *Lancet* medical journal in 1965 by a mother whose child had died after a routine tonsillectomy had a profound effect on both professional and public thinking. The letter read as follows:

My little girl Dawn was admitted to hospital for a tonsils and adenoids operation when she was three years and three weeks old. Up to then she had never been anywhere without me. I took Dawn to the hospital at 2.15 pm and was told to undress her and put her to bed. I was allowed to stay until 3 pm and told that I could return for visiting hour at 5-6 pm. When I returned at 5 o'clock I was told by the little boy in the next bed that Dawn had cried after me ever since I had left at 3 o'clock. I was told that I could not visit the next day because she was having the operation but they said that I could telephone. I telephoned a number of times the following day, and although Dawn was bleeding after the operation, I was not permitted to visit her. The next day I was told that I could visit her at 4 pm. I arrived at the ward at 3.50 pm and was told to wait because Dawn had collapsed. Shortly afterwards the ward sister came and told me that my dear Dawn had passed away at 4.15 pm. So you see, I couldn't go in to see Dawn even though she was dying. Other mothers who were on the ward told me that on the day of the operation, Dawn had returned to the ward and was crying constantly for me, and this I believe caused the bleeding. If this letter can help get another child united with her mother, please use it. After all, a nurse's skill cannot mend a child's broken heart, only a mother can do this because there is nothing in the world like a mother's love when a child is ill and upset.

This letter had a major impact on the thinking of both medical and nursing staff. Children are the only people on whose behalf other individuals may consent to medical procedures. Children are vulnerable, easily bewildered and frightened, and are unable to express their needs or defend their interests. The little girl described in the mother's letter was at the peak age for the effects of separation anxiety. Following this letter, a great relaxation in visiting policies took place, culminating in open visiting arrangements. The modern children's hospital is founded on two principles: parents must be allowed to visit and be present at all times, and the ward must be viewed as the child's temporary home.

PREPARING YOUR CHILD FOR HOSPITAL

Tell your child in advance that she is going into hospital. Reassure her that you will be there as much as possible and that she will be coming home again. For very young children aged between two and three years, two days' notice is sufficient. For children aged four to seven, a week's notice is advised so that the child can ponder on it and ask questions. In the case of older children, a frank discussion and involvement in the planning is recommended.

A child's understanding of illness is very much dependent on age and degree of maturity. Children often misunderstand the causes of illness and the reasons for medical and surgical treatments. Many young children think that painful procedures are a form of punishment. In one survey of children aged between five and thirteen years, all the five- to six-year-olds thought that treatment was punishment, those aged seven to ten years had some understanding of the purpose of treatment but remained very negative about any associated pain, while those over ten had a good comprehension of all aspects of hospital care. By getting your child to draw the body with the 'sore' part coloured in, it is possible to gain some insight into her understanding of the illness. (See also chapter on 'How Children Understand Illness'.)

Find out about the ward your child will be on and how long she is likely to be in hospital. Then discuss the details with her. Describe the beds, the ward and the different uniforms of the various members of the staff. Explain the everyday routines of hospital life: the child needs to know what time she will go to bed and get up, what the bathing and toilet arrangements will be, how she will occupy herself during the day. Explain about X-rays, injections, drips and blood tests. Tell her about the various people she will meet, including doctors, nurses, physiotherapists, radiographers, dieticians, teachers and play specialists.

In the case of an emergency admission, the time for preparation is considerably less, but it should still be possible to go quickly through most of the items already mentioned. Try to remain calm and in control as much as possible. If your distress and concern are too visible, your child may end up worrying about you as well as everything else.

What to bring to the hospital

Your child will need pyjamas, including a change. Bring toiletries, including toothbrush and toothpaste. Bring a favourite soft toy or blanket no matter how scruffy. Bring toys, games, paper and colouring materials to pass the time. In the case of a schoolgoing child, bring her schoolbooks and work copies.

COPING WITH HOSPITAL

How will your child cope with being in hospital?

The world that is perceived by a young child is narrow and confined to a few familiar faces, such as parents, grandparents, brothers, sisters, aunts, uncles and a few close neighbours. Admission to hospital is stressful because the child is confronted by a large number of strange people and surroundings that are new and frightening. The presence of a parent is the single most important factor in helping a child to cope with these anxieties. Simple, appropriate explanations about what is happening will help the child to cope. Watching familiar TV programmes and having favourite stories read to them is very helpful. The availability of school and play facilities will help to 'normalise' life. Children have a great capacity to adapt and adjust as long as they feel secure. Within a few days they will make friends with the other children, as well as with the nurses, doctors and the rest of the staff.

When visiting, remember to tell them about the other members of the family, as even young children quite often worry about what is happening at home in their absence. If pet animals are particularly missed, arrangements can sometimes be made for them to be brought to the reception area for a reunion with the child.

How will you cope with your child being in hospital?

Initially you will be very anxious and upset. If your child is undergoing surgery you will be anxiously awaiting the outcome. If your child has a medical problem you will be anxiously awaiting the results of tests and the response to treatment. At first you will probably want to be close to your child all the time. You may, however, feel bored and a little 'down' when the crisis has passed and the child is getting better. These feelings are natural and are to be expected. They are a result of stress, sleepless nights, irregular meals and the disruption of your normal everyday routines. Sitting beside a sick child's bed for hours on end, devoid of adult company, can be extremely monotonous. By its very nature a children's ward provides little in the way of distraction for a parent. There is a limit to how much television you can watch and how many books and magazines you can read. Also, you will be worried about the needs of the rest of the family. At times you may wonder whether your presence is really beneficial to your sick child. To avoid feeling like a captive parent, you need to be organised and to summon the support of your partner, relatives and friends. Get them to do 'sitting' sessions so that you can go home and have a bath, relax and get some fresh air. You will return in a much more positive frame of mind and will be in a better position to help and encourage your child.

Many children's hospitals have adopted 'care by parent' schemes. These were developed in the US in the early 1970s and were inspired by the feeling that families were the proper people to look after their own sick children. Under such schemes parents are permitted to participate and partake in the medical care of their children during the period in hospital. The tasks undertaken by parents include feeding at mealtimes, taking and charting temperature and pulse, and giving medication. These tasks help to reduce anxiety through involvement. In particular they help to reduce the feelings of loss of control that parents experience so readily when their child is being cared for by so many people in a strange environment. Studies have shown that children cared for by their parents in this manner cry less often, are more settled and are likely to be discharged more quickly.

The range of parental accommodation, although far from ideal, is steadily improving in Irish hospitals. To begin with, you may wish to sleep on a camp-bed beside your child on the ward. Later, when she is convalescent, you may wish for the peace and quiet of accommodation away from the ward.

Try, if possible, to be present for at least some of the doctors' ward rounds so that you can be brought up to date about your child's condition and what further medical measures are being considered. If you fully understand what is happening, you will find it easier to come to terms with your child's illness. Don't feel embarrassed if you find yourself asking the same questions repeatedly. This is very common and is a reflection of your anxiety.

The feelings of brothers and sisters

Children are deeply affected when a brother or sister is hospitalised with an illness. Most are unhappy and sad that their sibling is sick, and they find the physical separation upsetting. They are distressed by the inevitable disruption to family life. There may be anger due to decreased parental attention, which may in turn cause guilt.

The situation should be explained to them in simple terms. Every attempt must be made to preserve the normality of their lives. Arrangements should be made for them to visit their brother or sister in hospital. Involve them in the whole situation by getting them to make get-well cards, etc.

COMMON HOSPITAL PROCEDURES

The procedures that are frequently performed on children in hospital include intravenous drips and the taking of blood samples. Intravenous drips are often necessary if an ill child needs fluid, drugs or food, and can't take anything by mouth. The modern plastic 'cannulae' (tubes for inserting into blood vessels) are small enough to be used on even the youngest child or baby. The skin-prick is tiny, thus minimising the amount of pain experienced by the child. A special cream can be rubbed on the hand beforehand to further reduce pain. The cannula is quite secure in the vein and the child is free to move about. The doctor will try to site the drip in the left hand so that the right hand is free for drawing and writing, so do let the doctor know if your child is left-handed. If a parent is present during the procedure, the young child can be held sideways on the mother's lap. Explain to the child that the doctor will pinch her hand for a moment and that he/she will then put a big bandage on it.

Taking small samples of blood is the most common way of performing tests on sick children. The specific method used will depend on the age of your child. For babies under six months, a small heel-prick is frequently used. For older children the doctor will take the sample from the back of the hand or the front of the elbow.

Children undergoing complicated treatment for conditions such as cancer will require blood tests and other investigations such as lumbar punctures. Previously, many of these children developed 'needle phobia' which caused difficult psychological problems. Nowadays, it is the practice for all procedures on these children to be carried out under a light anaesthetic. The child experiences no pain and, more importantly, does not remember the unpleasant event.

Day-care surgery

Many of the surgical procedures performed on children can now be carried out on a day-care basis. The system is particularly suited to ear, nose and throat surgery, eye operations, undescended testicles, hernia repairs, etc. The child goes to the hospital in the morning, having fasted overnight. She is prepared for theatre, and following the surgery she returns to the day ward until fully recovered from the anaesthetic. After a final check-over, the child is then discharged home. Prior to discharge, arrangements are made for post-operative pain relief, change of dressings, etc. Day-care surgery has gained great popularity. It reduces to a minimum the distress to the child and the disruption to the family.

PLAY IN HOSPITAL

Play is a natural part of childhood and is necessary for normal, balanced development. To be allowed to play should be a right and not a privilege. Through the world of play a child explores her environment, acquires knowledge, expresses emotions, and copes with anxieties and worries. Play provides the child with an opportunity to act out the various experiences that she has had in the hospital. All modern hospitals recognise the necessity of providing play facilities for children. In the larger children's hospitals the play services are under the direction of qualified play specialists, whereas volunteers perform the role in smaller units.

On the ward, children are permitted to run about, play with toys and cycle tricycles. This atmosphere of 'chaos' is contrived rather than accidental. It is a recognition that the ward is the child's home. Children thrive and relax in this setting. The skill and challenge of paediatric nursing and medicine is the ability to administer high standards of care against this background.

The designated playroom provides children with the opportunity to play and meet other children. It is stocked with toys suitable for children of all ages. These supervised, organised play sessions take pressure off parents, both by giving them time off the ward and by helping them to play positively with their sick child.

In the case of a child confined completely to bed, the play specialist will visit the ward and provide appropriate play activities.

THE HOSPITAL SCHOOL

School is important for children during their stay in hospital. It allows them to continue their education throughout their illness and will minimise the adverse effects of being absent from their normal school. It is beneficial both to long-term patients and to those in hospital for just a few days. Children with chronic diseases may require frequent admissions throughout the year. For these, a planned curriculum can be arranged with the child's local school.

Every children's hospital in Ireland has its own school under the Department of Education. They are run by qualified teachers in a designated schoolroom within the hospital. They operate normal school hours, with the usual holiday periods.

In addition to the educational benefits, hospital school brings a degree of normality to the child's life. Sometimes it is the sickest children who work best and concentrate most, because this is the only aspect of their lives that they can control. School reassures them that they didn't have to give up everything when they became ill and that at least part of their lives is intact. The hospital school provides children with individual attention in a calm, non-threatening, non-competitive setting. Parents are encouraged to discuss their child's education with the teacher, so that specific learning difficulties can be assessed and appropriate advice given. In this way, in addition to the medical treatment, the child may benefit educationally during a stay in hospital.

ADOLESCENTS IN HOSPITAL

The ten to fifteen age group incorporates the transition from childhood through to adolescence. The special needs of adolescents in hospital are increasingly being recognised. These include privacy, facilities for recreation and education. Adolescents may feel uncomfortable and awkward on a children's ward, while an adult ward with mainly middle-aged patients is also unsuitable. Children's hospitals try to set aside an area for teenage patients where they can readily mix. Boredom can be a big problem for hospitalised adolescents with chronic conditions. Hospitals are sympathetic to the needs of these patients, in terms of wanting to stay up later to watch television, play computer games, read, etc. The accumulated evidence suggests that adolescents are best accommodated in purpose-designed wards, away from younger children and adults.

LONG-STAY OR FREQUENT HOSPITALISATION

Some children with chronic or complex conditions will require protracted or repeated hospital admissions, which will greatly disrupt both the child's life and that of her family. The problems are magnified when the family lives at a distance from the hospital. Considerable thought and planning are needed if the harmful psychological, emotional and educational effects are to be minimised. Flexibility is the key to overcoming many of these difficulties. Most of these children will not be undergoing constant treatment, so it will usually be possible for them to leave the hospital for an afternoon or perhaps go home for a weekend. These brief spells of normality are invaluable in maintaining a child's morale. An adjusted educational curriculum can be arranged through the hospital teacher. Hospital visits by friends and relatives need to be maintained in a regular and consistent manner. Experience has shown that hospital visits tend to fall away over time, leaving the child feeling isolated.

Many families find that having a sick child in hospital for a long period can cause financial problems. The costs incurred in travelling to and from the hospital can be substantial, and there are extra baby-minding expenses for the other children while the parents are at the hospital. In addition, the family income may be reduced due to the need to take time off work. The hospital authorities are aware of these difficulties and through the social work department can provide help and support.

The Association for the Welfare of Children in Hospital (AWCH) is actively involved in helping children and their families. The AWCH will arrange for a 'substitute mother' to visit your child. If you live a long way from the hospital, local branches of AWCH can be of help in meeting you from the train or bus and driving you to the hospital. It can also arrange overnight accommodation when needed.

WHEN YOUR CHILD COMES HOME

Write down instructions about diets, medications, dressings. Make a note of follow-up appointments. The days following discharge from hospital are a time of readjustment for both you and your child. Having been through a period of anxiety, fear and uncertainty, it can be difficult to re-establish normal routines at home. Your child may be more demanding and difficult to manage. Her appetite may be poor and her sleeping pattern may be disrupted. After a week, matters usually start returning to normal.

Useful address

Association for the Welfare of Children in Hospital (Ireland), 21 Ardagh Drive, Blackrock, Dublin. Tel. (01) 2889278.

Dr John F A Murphy FRCPI, DCH is Consultant Paediatrician at the National Maternity Hospital, Holles Street, Dublin, and Temple Street Children's Hospital, Dublin.

EAR, NOSE AND THROAT

MR TADHG O'DWYER

Disorders of the ear, nose and throat are the most common medical conditions in childhood, and the most frequent reason for surgery.

Many children go through a few years where they seem constantly to have an earache, a running nose or a sore throat. Tadhg O'Dwyer is a consultant ear, nose and throat specialist. He explains how parents can tell when their child has a mild problem that will clear with plenty of tender loving care, and when the child should be seen by a doctor.

THE EAR

The ear is divided into three main parts: the outer, middle and inner ear. The outer ear comprises the external ear and the ear canal, which leads to the ear-drum and the middle ear. The middle ear is composed of small bones which transmit sound to the inner ear. The inner ear is made up of the cochlea (the organ of hearing) and the labyrinth (the organ of balance). 'Hearing' involves the transfer of sound through the outer ear canal to the ear-drum. This sets the drum vibrating and the sound is transmitted via the small bones of the middle ear to the inner ear. Here the message is changed into electrical signals, which are transferred to the portion of the brain responsible for hearing.

INFECTIONS AND HEARING LOSS

There are two types of hearing loss or deafness: a) conductive hearing loss, where there is a blockage in the transmission of sound through the outer ear canal or, more commonly, through the middle ear, and b) inner ear or sensori-neural hearing loss, where there is an abnormality or damage to the nerves of the inner ear. Generally, where there is blockage in the outer ear canal or middle ear, the problem can be corrected. Damage to the inner ear, however, is permanent.

Hearing loss frequently results from an ear infection. Ear infections in children are extremely common and most children under the age of nine will have suffered at least once. A small proportion will suffer repeated infections.

Otitis media (middle ear infection)

A child with infection of the middle ear may have a severe pain in and around the ear, a loss of hearing and an increase in temperature, lasting one to two days. An earache should always be referred to your GP. If the infection is severe and is not treated with antibiotics, the ear-drum may perforate (rupture) and pus may be discharged. Once the ear-drum perforates, the pain subsides. At this stage it is important to start antibiotics, clear the pus from the ear and instil ear-drops. Generally the perforation in the ear-drum heals within two to three days, leaving no long-term damage.

Some children who suffer repeated infections may be left with a permanent perforation or hole in the ear-drum. This can also happen after a single severe infection, particularly if caused by measles or mumps, and hearing loss can be up to 30 per cent. The perforation is usually repaired by surgery after the child reaches the age of nine, and while hearing may be improved, it rarely returns to normal. The surgery will allow the child to resume swimming, which is normally 'out of bounds' to those with perforations, as contaminated water often gives rise to infection, with pain and discharge of pus.

Glue ear

With all ear infections, pus gathers in the middle ear, behind the ear-drum. The infection settles with the use of antibiotics and the pus clears. In some children it can take a prolonged period for the fluid to clear from the ear, and if it is present for more than twelve weeks, the condition is known as 'glue ear' — so-called because the fluid is often thick and sticky. It blocks the sound from passing through the middle ear, so there is an associated hearing loss. The hearing loss is often detected during the child's nine-month check-up, or at school. Alternatively, the parents may notice the child not responding when asked to do something, always having the television blaring, or being labelled inattentive at school.

The hearing loss associated with glue ear may vary from 10 to 30 per cent, and may affect one or both ears. When there is a bilateral loss (affecting both ears) of greater than 20 per cent, the child's speech development may be impaired, and this is likely to cause problems at school. The child may be labelled as having behavioural problems, but frequently this is due to frustration at not being able to detect what is being said.

Treatment of glue ear depends on whether one or both ears are affected, how long the fluid has been present and how much the child has suffered as a result. The only effective medical treatment is the use of antibiotics. A seven-day course of antibiotics may be prescribed or, alternatively, a nightly dose for three weeks.

Grommets

If antibiotic treatment is unsuccessful, the specialist may recommend the insertion of grommets. This surgery is usually performed under general anaesthetic on a day-patient basis. Grommets are tiny plastic tubes that are inserted into the ear-drum through a small incision in the lower part of the drum, after the fluid has been removed. They have a narrow segment in the middle, which allows them to sit in the drum, and they have a hollow centre so that air can enter the middle ear and prevent further fluid accumulation. They fall out of the ear-drums after six to nine months, and only rarely need to be removed surgically.

There are three main indications when grommets are used: a) bilateral hearing loss (greater than 20 per cent), where medical treatment has been unsuccessful; b) repeated ear infections; c) where complications such as damage to the ear-drum have begun.

Once the fluid is removed and the grommet is inserted, hearing usually returns to normal. In 70 per cent of children, grommets have to be inserted only once and the problem is cleared. However, a small percentage of children will require repeated grommet insertion before the problem resolves.

Parents often worry about the grommets falling out if the child falls, but this doesn't happen, even with the most robust of movements. Swimming with grommets is also a major parental concern, and some specialists refuse to allow children to swim with grommets in place. However, recent research suggests that it is only when contaminated water enters the ear under pressure, for example by jumping or diving into a pool, that the water passes through the grommet and the ear may become infected. It is therefore recommended that children with grommets wear ear-protectors (cotton wool dipped in Vaseline, or ear plugs) when swimming, in the bath or when having their hair washed.

INNER EAR HEARING LOSS

Hearing loss affects children differently from adults. It is easier for adults to compensate for a hearing loss, because they are already able to speak and understand language fully, than it is for a child whose hearing loss occurs before the ability to speak exists. It is also difficult to test children's hearing because they may not be able to cooperate with tests that are relatively easy for adults. Hearing tests for young children require special techniques and environments. For instance, their reactions to rattles and other sounds are often carefully observed. Rehabilitation is also different from that of adults, and continued education is very important because hearing loss also affects the child's learning ability. Simply providing a hearing-aid to a child with an inner ear hearing loss is not sufficient.

Inner ear hearing loss in children is usually present at birth. In 50 per cent of cases it is inherited from the parents and there is a family history of hearing loss. In the other 50 per cent of cases the mother may have developed an infection during pregnancy, for example rubella (German measles), or have encountered difficulties during delivery. Infections in the newborn baby, particularly meningitis, may also give rise to a hearing loss.

Early detection is vital if the child is to have normal speech. The most crucial time is the eighteen months to three-and-a-half year period, when the brain is most receptive to speech development. If a bilateral hearing loss (affecting both ears) is not detected until later, the child may never develop proper speech.

All children who are ill after birth, or who have to be looked after in an intensive care unit, are screened for a hearing loss. This group of children, as well as those with a family history of hearing loss, are ten times more likely to have hearing loss than normal babies. It is hoped that all children with an inner ear hearing loss will be detected by the age of one year.

Children with a mild hearing loss may require no treatment, but those with a moderate loss (30 to 50 per cent) will require a hearing-aid and special teaching to start with, although they will usually be able to attend a normal school later on. Children with severe to profound hearing loss (greater than 50 per cent) will have to attend a special school. Complete deafness in both ears is fortunately rare, but even in this group major advances are currently taking place, for example, the use of implant technology to place hearing-aid devices inside the inner ear (cochlear implant).

THE NOSE

Nasal blockage

Persistent nasal obstruction is a common complaint in children. It is often accompanied by the non-nasal symptoms of a dry, coated tongue, bad breath, snoring, mouth-breathing and post-nasal drip (fluid from the nose trickling down the throat). Common causes include:

- Enlarged adenoids: the adenoids, which are situated at the back of the nose, may become infected, causing a persistent infected nasal discharge. Adenoidectomy (removal of the adenoids) generally relieves the symptoms.

- A foreign body in the nose, for example, foam or other material: this usually gives rise to a persistent, dirty or foul-smelling nasal discharge. Removal of the object clears the problem.

- Septal deviation: the nasal septum is the partition that divides the nose into two passages. It may be displaced at birth or may be broken if the child falls or is hit on the nose. The problem is generally obvious when the nose is examined, and surgical correction is necessary in severe cases.

- Nasal allergy: this may be seasonal, where there is allergy to grass pollens, or perennial (all year round), caused by allergy to house-dust mites and dust. The child will sneeze and have a clear nasal discharge.

- Nasal polyps: these are grape-like structures that occur when the sinus lining becomes so swollen that it prolapses (falls down) into the nose. Nasal polyps are rare in children and occur most frequently in association with cystic fibrosis.

- Sinusitis: the sinuses are air-containing spaces within the bones of the face. When the mucous lining of the sinuses becomes infected, it is called sinusitis. It is estimated that 0.5 per cent of upper respiratory infections, which include colds, are complicated by acute sinusitis. On average, adults have two to five colds per year while children have six to eight, so it is not surprising that sinusitis is a common problem. It is frequently difficult to distinguish a simple cold from nasal allergy. However, in children with acute sinusitis the signs and symptoms of a cold are persistent. Nasal discharge and daytime coughs which continue beyond ten days and are not improving are the principal indicators. Less commonly, the child suffers from a high fever and persistent and infected nasal discharge. This is often associated with swelling of the eye and facial pain. In this case, immediate treatment is required. Chronic (ongoing) sinusitis should be suspected in children with persistent nasal discharge, nasal obstruction or cough, which has lasted more than one month. Examination and X-ray of the sinuses are the key to diagnosis.

  Treatment of acute sinusitis depends on the severity of the infection. In most cases, antibiotics are sufficient. However, if there is swelling around the eye, the child may be admitted to hospital for intravenous antibiotics. Those children with chronic sinusitis require careful evaluation, so as to eliminate an underlying problem such as tonsil or adenoidal infection or nasal allergy, which must be treated first. If the problem persists, surgery may be required.

Nosebleeds

Nosebleeds may occur at any age and at any time of the year. However, they occur more frequently in the winter months in association with colds, and in children between the ages of two and ten years. Nosebleeds in children are rarely associated with serious illness. They mostly occur in association with minor injury to the nasal lining, and they soon stop. When a nosebleed happens, pressure should be applied to the soft part of the nose until the bleeding has stopped. The head should be tilted forward, not backwards, as blood running down the back of the throat may cause the child to vomit. If the bleeding recurs frequently, then the child should see a doctor. A careful examination will usually reveal the cause. Blood tests may be necessary if there is a history of bleeding problems in the family. If the bleeding is from the front of the nose, cautery (burning) of the vessels may be required. This is a minor procedure which is performed under local anaesthesia, even in the young child.

THE THROAT

Sore throat is one of the most common problems the GP encounters. Four out of five cases are due to common respiratory viruses such as colds. Then the child may have a sore throat and be generally out of sorts. The child should be kept at home, given plenty to drink and allowed to eat as he feels like it.

Tonsils and adenoids

Some sore throats, however, are caused by a bacterial infection invading the tonsils. The tonsils and adenoids are part of the body's defence system against infection. They work by producing blood cells that combat infection, particularly during the first year of life. They increase in size during the first few years, but after the age of seven the adenoids begin to disappear, and the tonsils also shrink from puberty onwards.

A child with a bacterial infection will have a persistent fever, severe sore throat, and because of tonsillar enlargement may have difficulty swallowing. Tonsillitis is common in childhood, and may occur at any age, with a peak incidence at the age of five. If the symptoms are severe for more than twenty-four hours, or if there are spots of pus on the tonsils, your child should see a GP, who may prescribe antibiotics.

In some children infection develops deep in the core or centre of the tonsil and never clears fully. These children frequently have repeated infections, and in this event your doctor may advise that they be removed. During the 1930s tonsils and adenoids (T & A) surgery was the most common surgery performed worldwide. It was expected that the introduction of antibiotics would see the end of such surgery. However, this has not been the case, and it is still very common today, but it is usually reserved for those children with recurrent infections (four to five severe infections each year, requiring antibiotics). Removal of the tonsils and adenoids, even in a very young child, has never been shown to lead to increased infections after such surgery.

Extremely large tonsils and adenoids may impair normal breathing at night during sleep, and these children will snore loudly and can be heard outside their own room. In the more extreme cases, they may stop breathing for a few seconds at a time, and generally their sleep will be restless. They will get up frequently during the night to drink. They will eat poorly and appear not to be thriving. They will be lethargic during the day and have decreased stamina for athletic activities. Removal of the tonsils and adenoids in these children usually yields dramatic results.

The duration of stay in hospital after surgery is one to three days, but generally children are discharged the day after surgery. Complications are rare, the most serious being bleeding, which may occur either in the first few hours after surgery (primary haemorrhage), or a week later if the throat becomes infected (secondary haemorrhage). The risk of primary haemorrhage is one per thousand cases, while for secondary haemorrhage it is one per hundred cases. With primary haemorrhage, the child may need further surgical treatment to stop the bleeding, while with secondary haemorrhage the bleeding usually stops without treatment, but the child should always be brought back to hospital if bleeding occurs.

Hoarseness

Hoarseness is defined as a roughness in the quality of the voice resulting from an abnormality within the larynx (voice-box). The most common cause of hoarseness in childhood is vocal nodules. These are tiny swellings that occur on the edge of the vocal cords as a result of voice abuse (persistent shouting or screaming). Not all children who shout and scream develop vocal nodules, and frequently there are other contributory factors, such as irritation of the voice-box by smoke, noxious fumes from paint or pollution, chronic post-nasal drip, nasal allergy or sinusitis. Chronic cough or constant throat-clearing further damages already irritated vocal cords. Once the diagnosis of vocal nodules is made, the child is referred to a speech therapist who works to eliminate the vocal abuses and irritations and improves the child's voice function. With time and therapy, the nodules generally resolve without surgery.

Other causes of hoarseness are cysts and webs of the vocal cords, which are usually present at birth and have to be removed surgically. Children who require life-support in an intensive care unit, and therefore have a tube passing through the voice-box to the lungs, may develop scarring in the larynx, and once the tube is removed may have hoarseness or noisy breathing. Surgery may be required to correct the deformity.

Stridor

Stridor is a harsh sound that occurs during breathing and is caused by narrowing of the air passages. When it occurs in infancy and early childhood it can cause considerable concern to both parents and doctors. A child who has a high temperature and develops noisy breathing requires immediate hospitalisation. (See chapter on 'Breathing Problems'.)

Foreign bodies in the airway

A child who coughs and splutters after an object that was being held in its mouth disappears, is considered to have inhaled the object until proven otherwise. The most common age for this to occur is between the first and third year of life. After the initial coughing and spluttering the child may be well for days, even weeks. The most common objects aspirated into the lungs are peanuts, seeds, raisins and small plastic objects. Immediate assessment in hospital is required.

Foreign bodies in the oesophagus

Swallowing of foreign bodies is also common. Coins are most frequently swallowed, and if large they may become lodged in the oesophagus (gullet). In this event, they may have to be removed under general anaesthetic.

Mr Tadhg P O'Dwyer DLO, FRCSI, FRCS is Consultant Ear, Nose and Throat Specialist at The Children's Hospital, Temple Street, and Mater Hospital, Eccles Street, Dublin.

EYES

PROFESSOR LOUIS COLLUM

It is a wonderful moment when you first realise that your new baby is following you around the room with her eyes. This happens when she is about a month old. Sight develops quickly, and by her first birthday a child can see as well as an adult. Eyes are highly complex structures, capable of instantaneously receiving an ever-changing series of three-dimensional images. Louis Collum, Professor of Ophthalmology at the Royal Victoria Eye and Ear Hospital in Dublin, explains some of the conditions that can affect a child's eyes.

Sight is one of the most valued and important of our senses. Partial or total loss of sight is an enormous burden for anyone. However, with modern technology and efficient prevention and diagnosis, many of the conditions leading to sight impairment can now be treated.

Loss of sight is not as traumatic to a child as it is to an adult, who has already developed a particular lifestyle, both in terms of social activities and work. It is, however, a terrible experience for the parents of such a child. In Ireland, with good modern health care and education, the vast majority of childhood blinding conditions are now preventable.

THE EYE

Like the rest of the body, the eye has marvellous mechanisms for self-preservation. The eyeball sits in a bony cavity, surrounded by the nose, the cheek-bone and the brow, which protect it from knocks and blows. It is somewhat vulnerable, however, from the lateral (outer) side, the direction from which injuries are most likely to occur. Touch your own face and you will feel that the eyeball is protected only by layers of soft tissue on the lateral side! The wall of the eyeball itself is tough, consisting of the sclera (the white of the eye) and the cornea (the window of the eye). Any disturbance to the window of the eye will produce a blurring of vision. The cornea (window) acts like the glass in an ordinary window. If it becomes frosted, the inside of the eye does not receive the rays of light properly and vision becomes blurred.

From the front, the eye is also well protected, mainly by the eyelids, which automatically close at the least stimulus, such as a loud sound, a flash of light or any irritation of the skin or the lashes. In addition, the tears constantly wash the front of the eye, getting rid of all sorts of debris, which is present everywhere in the atmosphere. Tears also contain substances that can kill infectious agents. It is clear, therefore, that the eyeball can look after itself to a significant extent.

DETECTING EYE PROBLEMS

A baby does not see well immediately after birth, but her vision develops rapidly over the following two months, and the wandering eye movements that are commonplace in the first few months will usually have settled by six months. Parents should be able to notice obvious problems by then, such as 'turns' in the eye. In smaller babies the uncoordinated eye movements can be confusing.

Parents should observe what the baby is doing with her eyes. At an early stage a baby will fix her eyes on the mother, and will gaze at her while feeding. The ability to follow movement is a good sign that a baby's sight is developing normally.

In Ireland, babies' eyes are screened at birth, and then at intervals right through the primary school years. (The screening service is available free to all national schools.) At birth, the eyes are examined carefully so that early signs of disease can be detected. This is an important step in the prevention of serious eye problems at a later date. There are numerous congenital (present from birth) problems that can occur, for example, congenital glaucoma (pressure in the eye) and corneal dystrophies (haziness of the window of the eye), but luckily they are not common.

Parents with an eye problem such as retinitis pigmentosa (RP), which can lead to blindness, should have genetic counselling to establish the chances of their children developing the same condition.

The ongoing screening programme will usually pick up visual and structural abnormalities, including squints and congenital diseases, such as glaucoma or cataract, as well as early signs of some systemic (general) diseases. This is an invaluable service and one all children should avail of. If a problem with sight is developing, the sooner it is dealt with, the better.

Most family doctors automatically do some assessment of the eyes when children are brought to them for any reason. They can deal with minor problems, but will usually refer anything more serious to a specialist.

CONGENITAL EYE DISORDERS

Squint

A squint (also known as a cast, a turn or a stare) is where one eye appears to be directed inwards towards the nose, or outwards. Because a baby's eye movements are somewhat erratic, it is not always easy to notice a squint at an early age. However, if you are worried that your child may have a squint, it is of the utmost importance that she be assessed by a doctor at the earliest possible moment. A baby is never too young for assessment where a squint is suspected. There are a number of reasons for this.

Firstly, if a baby is turning an eye, the chances are that she will not use that eye and it may become amblyopic (lazy). The visual pathways to the brain will not develop and the child will have defective sight for life.

Secondly, there may be disease inside an eye that interferes with the ability of the back of the eye to perceive images. This will result in the eye slipping out of position. Generally, sight is the stimulus for an eye to remain straight, and if the sight is not getting through, the eye becomes like a ship without an anchor and will wander out of place. Abnormalities inside the eye that can result in a squint include a haemorrhage, a developmental problem, a cataract (an opaque lens), and very occasionally a tumour.

Sometimes parents look at their children and are certain they have a squint. This may not always be the case. The child appears to have a squint because of a condition called 'epicanthus', where the bridge of the nose is flat and there is a fold of skin running from the upper lid to the lower lid, at the inner corner of the eye. This is not a problem, as the bridge of the nose will usually build up as the child gets older and the so-called squint will no longer be present. However, where there is any suspicion at all, the child should be fully assessed.

A straightforward squint should be treated from a very early stage. Squints are dealt with by putting a patch over the 'good eye' or by glasses, which may help prevent the development of amblyopia (laziness). Surgery (which is usually done later than the baby stage) may be required to improve sight or for reasons of appearance. Orthoptic treatment (eye exercises) can also be helpful.

Cataract

Cataract is a condition whereby the lens is either partially or completely opaque, preventing images from getting to the back of the eye, and leading to blurring or total loss of vision. Congenital (from birth) cataract should be dealt with when the baby is still very young, even less than six weeks old. If the operation is deferred, the visual pathways will not develop, as the major part of visual development occurs at a very early stage.

Cataract surgery consists of removing the lens, which is opaque, and inserting a 'plastic' lens inside the eye. While there are some technical and optical problems associated with this operation, it does offer children with congenital cataracts a good chance of normal vision.

Toxoplasmosis and toxocariasis

These are rare conditions that can affect the back of the eye and damage the sight.

If a pregnant woman is infected by the toxoplasmosis protozoa (worm), which can happen through eating undercooked meat from an infected animal, or by picking up the worm from cats' faeces, her baby's eyes may in turn be damaged. Toxocariasis is a related infection that is caused by a parasitic worm found in the intestines of dogs. Both these organisms are present quite commonly in areas that have been fouled by dogs and cats. Animals should not be exercised or let loose where small children play, because of the danger that the animals' droppings will contaminate sand pits, etc. As children put things in their mouths, they can easily pick up such infections.

Toxoplasmosis can be treated reasonably effectively, though depending on where it is sited at the back of the eye, significant damage can result. The treatment for toxocariasis is not so satisfactory, and the child's sight may be permanently affected.

Viral infections

Viral infections in the mother can harm a foetus. Rubella (German measles), for example, if contracted during the early stages of pregnancy, can affect the child's cornea (window of the eye), can cause cataract and can produce major changes at the back of the eye, some of which may be difficult to treat.

EYE INFECTIONS

Children get infections easily in many parts of the body, and the eye is no exception.

Stye

A stye is an infection of the lash follicle (root). Styes are purely superficial infections, which are treatable by antibiotics and by bathing the eyelid with warm water. If they are occur frequently, they may be a sign that the child is diabetic. Styes are commonly associated with greasy skins, and with conditions such as eczema and psoriasis. (See chapter on 'Skin Conditions'.)

Sticky eyes

Some babies are born with sticky, watery eyes, or they may acquire the condition soon after birth. This is due to a blocked tear duct. The tear duct is a small duct running from the inner corner of the eye into the nose, and is essential for the drainage of fluid away from the eye. In some babies the tear duct does not open fully at birth, and this predisposes them to infection. The condition often responds to careful cleaning of the eyes with cotton wool dipped in cooled, previously boiled water, but sometimes antibiotics are required. Very occasionally, a small operation may be necessary to free the duct. It is usually not a serious problem.

Conjunctivitis

'Conjunctivitis' is a fairly non-specific term and can indicate a number of conditions. It simply means 'red eye'.

Childhood infections such as measles, mumps and chicken-pox are often accompanied by inflammation (redness) of the eyes and a watery discharge. This type of conjunctivitis is usually not serious. It will normally clear up spontaneously after a few days, but it may require local treatment with drops or ointment.

Conjunctivitis due to bacterial organisms is, however, much more common. It frequently looks worse than it is, with a yellow or green discharge which causes the lashes to be matted together in the mornings. Again it is usually not a serious condition and can be treated by the family doctor with an antibiotic.

Some red eyes are due to foreign bodies lodged in the cornea or concealed under the lids. Thorough examination (with or without anaesthesia) should reveal these, and they are easily removed by the doctor.

Corneal ulcers

Not all red discharging eyes in children are totally harmless. Ulcers, for example, may develop on the cornea (window of the eye). In this case the eye will be sore as well as red, but the discharge will not be quite so copious. Care must be exercised in this instance, as corneal ulcers can lead to a significant reduction in vision. It is sometimes necessary to examine the child under anaesthesia in order to make an absolute diagnosis. Corneal ulcers may be caused by viruses such as *Herpes simplex* (the cold sore virus), as well as by bacterial infection.

EYE INJURIES

Perhaps the most tragic of all occurrences in children are eye injuries. Many of these are preventable, being caused by carelessness in the home and elsewhere. These accidents are not as rare as might be imagined. Children are inquisitive and tend to investigate all sorts of nooks and crannies. It is vital that dangerous implements such as knives, forks and scissors should not be left lying around. Toys should be safe and anything with sharp edges and wires should be avoided, whatever age the child is. The popularity and increased use of fireworks, particularly at

Hallowe'en, has introduced an additional risk. Fireworks cause numerous eye injuries every year, some involving complete loss of sight. If fireworks must be used, they should be strictly supervised by an adult — even then they are still dangerous.

SHORTSIGHTEDNESS

Myopia (short sight) is a condition that commonly develops in later childhood. Usually parents or teachers will notice the child 'squinting' (narrowing her eyelids together) or moving closer in order to see the television or blackboard. This is an attempt to focus the rays of light onto the back of the eyeball, which has become too long as the child has grown. This is a simple condition and the child merely needs spectacles to correct it.

Keratoconus, also called conical cornea, is a more serious condition. The shape of the front of the eye becomes abnormal; instead of being nicely rounded, the cornea (window) becomes somewhat pointed. This results in the inability of rays of light to focus on the back of the eye, thereby affecting the sight. It is frequently associated with allergic problems, such as asthma, eczema and hayfever, and is also commonly found in children with Down's Syndrome. In the early stages, contact lenses may remedy the problem, but some sufferers will require corneal transplantation, which is a very successful operation.

Useful addresses

RP Ireland (Retinitis Pigmentosa Society), 45a Whitworth Road, Drumcondra, Dublin 9. Tel. (01) 8307955.
Irish Fight for Sight, 4 Parnell Street, Waterford. Tel. (051) 78088.

Professor L M T Collum FRCS, FRCSI, FRC Ophth is Professor of Opthalmology at the Royal College of Surgeons in Ireland and the Royal Victoria Eye and Ear Hospital, Dublin.

FEEDING YOUR CHILD

SINÉAD FEEHAN

When we feed our children we are not only providing them with the nourishment they need to grow up strong and healthy, we are also influencing their taste and appreciation of food, and helping them develop good eating habits for later life.

Clinical nutritionist/dietitian Sinéad Feehan gives advice on feeding throughout childhood, including breast and bottlefeeding, how to cope with a toddler's food fads, and how to make sure an adolescent is eating sensibly.

BREASTFEEDING

Breastfeeding is undoubtedly the most desirable form of feeding for infants. A mother's own milk will provide her baby with all the nutrients and energy it requires for growth and development, in an easily digestible, easily absorbed form.

Breast milk is a remarkably variable food. Its composition changes during the breastfeeding period to meet the constantly changing needs of the growing baby. It has special properties that help to give the baby immunity from infection, especially during the first few weeks of life when the infant is quite vulnerable. These properties may also help reduce the child's chances of developing conditions such as eczema, asthma and food intolerance later in life. Breastfeeding also has many practical benefits. Breast milk is readily available at all times, costs nothing, and requires no preparation or special equipment.

Breastfed babies should be fed 'on demand' — the more frequently the baby suckles the more milk will be produced. Unfortunately mothers often stop breastfeeding because they believe that they are not producing enough milk. But if a baby who seems hungry between feeds is put to the breast more often, the milk supply will increase. In the first few weeks of life breastfed babies tend to need short but frequent feeds. With time, however, a feeding pattern will emerge, with the baby feeding longer at each breast, and longer gaps between feeds. By two to three weeks many infants will feed for fifteen to twenty minutes from each breast. Additional fluids, 'complementary' or 'top-up' feeds should not be given. They are unnecessary and can interfere with the establishment of successful breastfeeding.

Coping with a new baby and trying to breastfeed can be exhausting for the new mother, so it is important that she gets as much rest as possible. Support and help from her partner, friends and family, with duties such as housework, shopping and changing nappies, is essential and offers should never be refused. It is also very important that breastfeeding mums eat a healthy and varied diet, with adequate fluids, to help meet their increased nutritional requirements.

Despite the uniqueness of breast milk and the many advantages of breastfeeding, the incidence of breastfeeding in Ireland is low. It is estimated that only about a quarter of Irish babies are breastfed. (See 'Breastfeeding techniques', p46.)

BOTTLEFEEDING

Bottlefeeding is generally a safe and satisfactory alternative to breastfeeding, provided an approved infant formula is used. There is a wide range of formulated feeds available containing all the nutrients required for growth during the first six months of life.

Infant formula

Most formula milks are based on cow's milk that has been greatly modified to ensure its suitability for young infants and to mimic human milk as closely as possible. They fall into two categories:

1) Whey-based formula, such as Aptamil, Nutrilon Premium, Ostermilk and SMA Gold Cap.

2) Casein-based formula, such as Milumil, Nutrilon Plus, Ostermilk Two and SMA White Cap.

Although there is no firm evidence upon which to base a choice of one particular brand over another, a whey-based formula would appear to be more suitable for newborn babies as its protein composition is closer to that of human milk, while the casein-based formula is generally given to 'hungrier' infants. However, they are all satisfactory feeds and suitable for all infants. Babies should never be given ordinary cow's milk, evaporated milk, goat's milk or unmodified soya milk.

Making up feeds

It is essential to follow the manufacturer's instructions carefully when making up feeds. Adding an extra scoop of formula, cereals or rusks to an infant's bottle could cause high salt levels, leading to dehydration or damage to the kidneys. Over-concentrated feeds could also make the baby fat, which can lead to long-term obesity. Over-diluting feeds, on the other hand, could result in the infant failing to thrive.

Bottles and other feeding equipment must be cleaned, sterilised and stored carefully to reduce the risk of contaminating feeds with bacteria.

How much feed?

Bottlefed infants should be fed on demand in much the same way as breastfed infants, allowing them to regulate their own volume of intake. It is important to remember that all babies differ in their needs, so the amount of milk (breast or bottle) taken will vary from baby to baby according to weight, activity, growth rate and appetite. If a baby is gaining weight appropriately in relation to its length, parents can be assured that their child is feeding adequately. Generally speaking, by three to four weeks a baby will be taking two to three ounces of milk per pound of bodyweight per day. If the baby takes less than one ounce per pound per day, then it is important to seek the advice of your doctor.

Extra drinks

Extra drinks of water or fruit juice should not generally be encouraged, for either breastfed or bottlefed babies, particularly during the early weeks of life, as this could interfere with the establishment of feeding. Breastfed babies rarely need extra drinks. However, if a bottlefed baby appears thirsty between feeds or becomes constipated, small quantities of cooled boiled water could be offered. Baby drinks and fruit juices contain glucose or fructose, and although these are less harmful than sucrose (sugar), they can damage the baby's teeth. They should be used as little as possible and only if well diluted.

Wind and posseting (milk regurgitation)

Bottlefed babies tend to take in more air than breastfed babies and can, as a result, suffer from the discomfort of wind and/or milk regurgitation during or after a feed. These are generally not serious problems, but they can be distressing for both baby and parents. Check the teat to make sure that the hole is neither too large nor too small. Hold the bottle up so that the teat does not empty, causing the baby to suck in air. Gently wind the baby at intervals during feeding.

Switching feeds

Parents often feel that problems such as wind, colic and posseting are due to a 'feed intolerance' or 'allergy', and change to a different brand of feed. Sometimes they try a number of different feeds without success. Although switching feeds probably doesn't do any harm, it is usually unnecessary. You should never change a baby's feed before first checking your feeding technique, the teat size, feed volume and frequency.

Cow's milk

Breast or formula milks are the only milks suitable for infants under six months. At the six-month stage, parents are often tempted to switch over to using cow's milk for reasons of convenience and/or cost. Cow's milk, however, is not recommended before the age of twelve months. It contains too much salt (which the young child's kidneys cannot handle) and it is too low in most vitamins and minerals, particularly iron. A child should be kept on breast or formula milk until he is at least one year old and consuming a varied diet. A mother who chooses to breastfeed her baby for longer than the first year should make sure that both she and the baby are getting an adequate diet.

Follow-on milk

A follow-on milk such as Progress, Junior Milk, or Step-Up may be used after six months. These have a higher protein and salt content than normal formulae so they are unsuitable for younger babies. One advantage of follow-on milks is their high iron content. However, from six months onwards milk should not be the main source of iron in a child's diet. It should be coming from iron-rich solid foods such as meat. Follow-on milks, therefore, have no real advantage over continued breastfeeding or using a normal formula.

Soya formula

Soya formula is made from vegetable oils and protein instead of cow's milk. Like the standard formula it contains adequate amounts of iron and vitamins, but is more expensive. The principal reason for using a soya formula is allergy to cow's milk protein, which is very uncommon. Signs of allergy include severe irritability, poor weight gain, vomiting and rash.

WEANING

Weaning a baby onto solids should be a gradual process over several weeks and months, starting somewhere between three and six months. Weaning begins when breast or formula milk ceases to be adequate as the sole source of nutrition for the growing infant.

From twelve weeks the swallowing reflex is developed enough to enable an infant to take puréed foods. Solids should never be given before three months as this could increase the risk of developing infections, allergies, coeliac disease (disease of the intestines) or obesity. On the other hand, failure to give a child solids by six months could result in difficulties in learning to chew and in the child being reluctant to accept solids when they are eventually given.

First weaning foods

The first food offered to an infant should be very smooth, bland to taste and gluten-free, for example, puréed baby rice mixed with breast or formula milk. Puréed or sieved fruit or vegetables such as pear, apple, carrot and potato are equally acceptable for first tastes.

Initially one or two teaspoons should be offered before a normal breast or bottle feed. However, very hungry babies may cope with solid foods more easily after some milk has been offered to take the edge off their hunger.

With time, the quantity and number of solid feeds taken should gradually increase. To add variety and to improve iron intake, small amounts of puréed red meat or chicken should be given.

Before six months, eggs, dairy products (cow's milk, cheese and yoghurts), and foods containing gluten (bread, rusks and wheat-based cereals such as Weetabix), should not be given, because of their association with food allergy and coeliac disease.

By six months

By six months babies should be taking three small spoonfeeds daily. Normal family and homecooked foods (without added salt or sugar) are preferable to commercial baby foods as they are cheaper, parents know what the ingredients are, and the baby will get used to eating like the rest of the family more quickly.

The volume of milk (breast or bottle) taken by the child will gradually decrease as the quantity of solid foods increases. However, milk will continue to be a very important part of the child's diet throughout the first year of its life.

From six months to one year

From six months a baby will gradually learn to cope with food that is lumpier in texture. Moving from puréed to mashed or minced foods will encourage the child to chew and to use his mouth and tongue, which will in turn help with teething and speech. Continuing to introduce new foods will enable the child to get used to new tastes and textures, while ensuring a good diet. (See 'Weaning-Food Guide' below.)

At this stage babies will begin to take an interest in feeding themselves. Although messy, self-feeding should be encouraged. Mealtimes, as well as being a time for learning, should be a time for fun!

As the ability to grasp and pick up foods develops, babies should be offered finger foods, such as small chunks of cheese, fingers of toast, pieces of apple or pear. However, a child should never be left alone with any food, in case of choking. A beaker or cup for drinking can be introduced from six to seven months.

Sugar

It is important not to add sugar to a child's food, nor to give snacks of biscuits and chocolate, as sugar is a major cause of tooth decay. Frequent drinks of fruit juice, squashes and fizzy drinks are also harmful to the teeth. More suitable drinks to offer include boiled, cooled water, well-diluted juices or a sugar-free squash.

WEANING-FOOD GUIDE

From three to four months

Try: Vegetable purées — carrot, turnip, potato
       Fruit purées — apple, pear, banana
       Pure baby rice

Up to six months

Try: Meat purées — beef, lamb, chicken
       Fish — flaked and puréed
       Wider variety of vegetables — broccoli, cauliflower, beans
       Fruit — peach and plums

Avoid: Milk (other than breast or formula), cheese, yoghurt, eggs
       Wheat-based foods — bread, rusks, cereals
       Sugar, salt, nuts

From six months

Try: Cheese, yoghurt, fromage frais
        Wheat-based cereals — Weetabix, Branflakes
        Bread, rusks, crackers
        Citrus fruits — oranges, mandarins
        Minced meat and poultry
        Mashed potatoes and vegetables

THE TODDLER AND PRE-SCHOOL YEARS

From one year, most babies, now toddlers, should happily eat normal family foods presented in a suitable and attractive form. Offering toddlers a good variety, from a range of nutrient-rich foods such as milk, meat, poultry, fish, cheese, yoghurt, bread, cereals, fruit and vegetables, will help ensure an adequate intake of all the nutrients and energy required for further growth and development. (See 'Four Food Groups', p120.)

Fat is an important source of energy for growing children, so it is better to give them full-fat milk, cheese and yoghurts, rather than the 'low fat' or 'diet' variety. The fat in such foods is also a source of vitamins A and D.

As children have small appetites and tend to eat small meals, offering nutritious snacks such as pieces of fruit, cheese, crackers and small sandwiches are a good way of supplementing their meals and improving their overall nutritional intake. Leaving long gaps between meals, without anything to eat, can lead to hunger, bad temper and constant demands for biscuits, crisps and sweets.

Vitamin supplements

Parents often wonder if they should be giving their child extra vitamins and minerals in the form of a supplement. These are usually unnecessary — a child will get all the vitamins and minerals he needs from a healthy diet made up of a variety of foods.

Iron-deficiency anaemia

Iron-deficiency anaemia is a very common problem amongst Irish infants and toddlers. It can cause the child to be uninterested in food, lethargic, to lose weight, and fail to thrive.

Typically, the diets of iron-deficient toddlers consist mainly of bread, yoghurts, tea and large volumes of cow's milk. This sort of diet is low in iron and in vitamin C (which aids iron absorption from foods).

Iron deficiency can be prevented by including red meats, green leafy vegetables and iron-fortified breakfast cereals, together with a combination of foods containing vitamin C, such as fruit, fruit juice, vegetables and salads, in the weaning and toddler diet.

Constipation

Constipation can be a problem for some children, particularly from the age of two. Instead of giving laxatives, the child's diet should be adjusted to help achieve a regular bowel habit.

1) Make sure the child has regular meals and snacks.

2) Gradually increase the child's fibre intake by encouraging him to eat wholemeal bread, fibre-rich cereals such as Weetabix, fruit and vegetables.

3) Give plenty of fluids, such as water, sugar-free squash and diluted fruit juices, throughout the day.

Food fads

Many toddlers go through phases of food fads or strikes, such as eating very little of anything; eating well but from a very limited range of foods; or preferring peculiar food combinations (such as baked beans and cornflakes). Such phases can cause a lot of anxiety and frustration in parents. Mealtimes frequently turn into a battle, with the parents being the losers!

Like adults, children's appetites vary from day to day. They have their likes and dislikes, which keep changing. It is part of their normal development to experiment with food, and although they may appear to be eating very little, or eating a bizarre diet, children do eventually sort out their eating habits. They don't starve themselves!

The best way to deal with food fads is to ignore the whole matter (which is often easier said than done). Generally, such strikes don't last very long, and providing the child is gaining weight and thriving, parents need not worry.

Having regular times for meals, eating at the table with the rest of the family, making food look interesting and colourful, may help the situation. Food that is refused should be removed without comment. The strong impulse to offer biscuits or sweet foods as an alternative should be resisted. A relaxed attitude on the part of parents will help resolve the problem more quickly.

THE PRIMARY SCHOOL YEARS

The primary school child has a continuing need for a nourishing diet, which can be provided with a variety of foods throughout the day. (See 'Four Food Groups', p120.) When a child begins school, several lifestyle and eating-pattern changes occur. Getting to school on time can interfere with breakfast, while the midday meal and snacks are frequently taken at school.

Nutritional problems, such as iron-deficiency anaemia, poor growth, dental disease and obesity, can arise if meals are constantly missed or if snacks and school lunches consist of poor-quality foods, such as crisps, biscuits, chocolate bars and sugary drinks. Ensuring that a child does not miss meals, especially breakfast, and providing healthy packed lunches and snacks for school, will help safeguard against such problems.

HEALTHY LUNCHBOX IDEAS

Sandwiches
Bread, baps, rolls (wholemeal and white) with various fillings:
cheese & tomato
egg salad
chicken & sweetcorn
ham & lettuce

bacon, lettuce and tomato
tuna fish & celery

Snacks
fresh fruit
yoghurts
fromage frais
dried fruit
fruit & nut mix
muesli crunch bar

Drinks
milk
unsweetened fruit juice
sugar-free squash

ADOLESCENCE

Adolescence is the transitional period between childhood and adulthood, during which rapid psychological, social, intellectual and physical changes occur. Because of the rapid growth spurt that occurs at this time, energy and nutrient requirements are greatly increased. However, during adolescence, eating habits may become erratic, with appetites and intakes varying from day to day, while convenience or 'fast foods' become increasingly popular. Parents need a lot of patience, tact and understanding so that their teenager is gently steered towards a pattern of sensible eating.

Energy

Energy requirements are particularly high in adolescent boys, who may need to consume as much as 3000 to 4000 calories a day — twice as much as their parents. For many, frequent snacks, in addition to substantial meals, are the only way to obtain sufficient energy.

Iron

Iron requirements increase in girls with the onset of menstruation. Iron-deficiency anaemia is not uncommon in this age group, particularly if their dietary intake of iron is inadequate. This can be a problem particularly for girls who decide to become vegetarian and start omitting animal products (such as red meats) from their diet without having suitable alternatives.

Vegetarians need to eat more wholegrain cereals, pulses (peas, beans, lentils), dried fruit and nuts. To aid the absorption of iron from these foods, vitamin C food (fruit, fruit juice, vegetables, salad) should be eaten at the same time.

Calcium

Calcium requirements also increase during adolescence because this is a time of rapid bone growth and development. Hence the importance of milk, cheese and yoghurt in the teenager's diet. Other sources of calcium include tinned sardines and salmon (including the bones), bread, almonds, and green vegetables such as broccoli.

Food fads and slimming

Food faddism, based on misconceptions about food, may lead to poor food choice and inadequate diets. Teenage girls in particular, and some boys, who become overconcerned about their weight, can turn to very restrictive slimming methods to lose weight. Fortunately, most fads are short-term. However, if the weight loss is rapid, professional help should be sought quickly. (See also chapter on 'Anorexia and Bulimia'.)

Dietary advice

Adolescents should be educated on the importance of nutrition and health, and of eating a variety of foods to meet their nutritional requirements. While the general principles of a healthy diet apply to this age group too, parents must take into account the adolescent's lifestyle. So, for teenagers who prefer to 'eat on the run', it may be better to provide frequent nutritious snacks, incorporating the occasional convenience or take-away foods, rather than insisting on regular 'proper' meals.

FOUR FOOD GROUPS

Food	Meat & alternatives	Milk products	Fruit & veg	Potato & cereals
Serving sizes	2oz (57g) lean meat	⅓ pint milk	1 fresh fruit	1 slice bread
	3oz (85g) fish	1 yoghurt	1 portion veg	1 potato
	2oz (57g) poultry	1oz (28g)	1 portion salad	Bowl cereal
	2oz (57g) hard cheese	cheese (cheddar)	Glass fruit juice	2 tbsp rice/pasta
	2 eggs		Bowl stewed fruit	
	6 tbsp beans/peas			
Main nutrients	Protein, iron	Calcium	Vitamins C & A	Energy
	B vitamins	Protein	Folic acid	B vitamins
		Vitamin A	Fibre	Minerals
Daily serving				
Child:	2	3	4	4
Teenager:	2	5	4	6+

Useful address

La Leche League of Ireland (Breastfeeding Help and Information), PO Box 1280, Raheny, Dublin 5.

Sinéad Feehan BSc is Senior Clinical Nutritionist/Dietitian at the National Children's Hospital, Harcourt Street, Dublin.

FITS, FAINTS AND FUNNY SPELLS

DR JOE McMENAMIN

If your child has any kind of fit, faint or funny spell, you are likely to be extremely concerned. Unconsciousness, even when it lasts only for a few minutes, can be very worrying.

Dr Joe McMenamin, who is a consultant paediatric neurologist, outlines the many types of seizures that can affect the brain, from the more serious forms of epilepsy to the more common occurrences such as daydreaming and febrile convulsions.

EPILEPTIC SEIZURES

The brain is the control centre for the nervous system. It controls all voluntary functions, walking, talking, seeing, hearing and communicating with the world outside. It does this by transmitting and receiving electrical signals along biological wires called nerves. The brain is like a computer, and as with a computer, it can suddenly malfunction. If this happens, a sudden discharge of brain electricity may occur and result in loss of consciousness, change of behaviour or involuntary movements called seizures. The diagnosis of epilepsy is usually based on the history of recurring seizures and a brain-wave test known as an electroencephalogram or EEG, which measures brain electricity. When epilepsy is present the excessive electrical discharges are recorded and this helps the doctor to decide on the type of epilepsy and the treatment required.

Drugs used in the treatment of epilepsy include Tegretol, Epilim, Zarontin and Epanutin. Unlike adults, most children grow out of their epilepsy and only require medication for a few years. Only a very small number of children fail to respond to medication, and in such cases brain surgery may be considered. Approximately 0.5 per cent of the Irish population have epilepsy, and the majority have their first seizure in childhood. There are many different types of epilepsy, but some are more common than others. Certain varieties are hereditary or genetic, and occasionally a severe head injury or underlying brain disease may be the cause, but in the vast majority of children there is no known cause or other underlying condition present.

'Grand mal' or 'tonic-clonic' seizures

'Grand mal' (French for 'big seizure') is the common term for a tonic-clonic seizure, the type of seizure that most people equate with epilepsy. Typically, the attack begins with a sudden loss of consciousness and falling to the ground. The body stiffens for fifteen to thirty seconds (tonic phase), and this is usually followed by jerking of the trunk and limbs (clonic phase), which can last for a variable period of time. During this type of seizure the child may have difficulty breathing and become cyanosed (blue), particularly around the lips, and the bladder and bowel may empty. Following the seizure, drowsiness or more often a deep sleep ensues, which may last hours.

Treatment of the seizure consists of placing the child in the recovery position, i.e. on her side, removing tight clothing and any objects in the mouth that might obstruct the airway and breathing. It is imperative not to put anything into the mouth. There is no need to be concerned about tongue-swallowing causing airway obstruction. Putting objects such as a spoon into the mouth to prevent swallowing of the tongue may induce vomiting or some other complication which could be dangerous. It is best to let the seizure take its course.

Like most forms of epileptic seizures, tonic-clonic seizures occur more often in the morning, sometimes before waking, and an EEG test done at this time usually shows bursts of electrical discharges from both sides of the brain. Most young people with tonic-clonic seizures have no other medical or neurological problems. Up to 25 per cent will have a family history of similar convulsions, indicating that the cause is genetic. Treatment of recurring tonic-clonic seizures involves taking anti-epileptic medication regularly, usually twice daily.

'Petit mal' or absence seizures

'Petit mal' (French for 'small seizure') or absence seizures typically consist of a sudden cessation of activity, blank staring, with a characteristic vacant facial expression, often accompanied by rhythmic flickering of the eyelids. In contrast to tonic-clonic seizures, the child never falls down, and the episodes last less than fifteen seconds, with instantaneous recovery. Usually the child has no memory of events that occurred during the seizure and will resume all activities immediately afterwards as if nothing happened. Attacks can occur frequently and can vary from just a few each day to hundreds. They tend to occur in the morning and afternoon, particularly if the child is tired. Frequent absence seizures during classroom hours will interfere with the child's education.

The doctor will diagnose absence seizures by simply having the child hyperventilate or overbreathe, a procedure that will bring on an attack. Further confirmation can be obtained by doing an EEG test. Treatment involves taking anti-epileptic medication such as Zarontin or Epilim, to which most children with simple absences will respond. Absence seizures occur mostly in children between the ages of five and twelve years, and most grow out of this type of epilepsy. Up to 25 per cent of cases will have a family history of similar seizures. A small number of children with absence epilepsy will also suffer from major tonic-clonic seizures.

Partial seizures

Grand mal and petit mal seizures are generalised seizures because they are caused by abnormal electrical discharges within the whole brain. In partial seizures the abnormal electrical activity arises from a localised area of the brain, for example, the temporal lobe on the side of the brain.

Symptoms in partial seizures vary quite a lot, and differ from generalised seizures in a number of ways. In partial seizures there is often an aura or warning prior to the onset of the episode. This may consist of a feeling of fear or an hallucination, such as hearing a sound that is not present, or more commonly a sensation of discomfort in the tummy, rising up into the throat. Symptoms depend on the part of the brain involved. Partial seizures from the temporal lobe often begin with a sensation of fear, quickly followed by altered awareness or consciousness, often accompanied by staring, involuntary lip smacking, chewing or swallowing movements, or aimless picking at clothes with the fingers. The seizure may be confined to this type of symptom or may evolve into jerking of the limbs, often involving only one side of the body. Recovery is gradual, and after the seizure the child is often confused and disorientated and wishes to sleep.

Partial seizures are not always associated with impaired consciousness and the child may be fully alert throughout the episode and able to relate all of the symptoms experienced. In this situation they are called simple partial seizures, and where consciousness is impaired or lost they are called complex partial seizures. Partial seizures are more likely to occur when the susceptible child is tired, stressed or has an infectious disease, particularly with fever. In addition to the EEG test, some form of brain-imaging test such as a CAT (Computerised Axial Tomography) scan or MRI (Magnetic Resonance Imaging) scan will be required. Treatment consists of taking anti-epileptic medication such as Tegretol, Epilim and Epanutin. If seizures are completely controlled by drug therapy, the long-term outlook is very good. Many children will eventually come off medication and will have no further problems. Some, however, and particularly those who do not respond well to treatment, will need long-term medication. A small number of children with partial seizures may be considered suitable candidates for epilepsy surgery.

SEIZURES AND TURNS THAT ARE NOT EPILEPSY

Fainting seizures

Most people are familiar with or have witnessed a typical fainting episode. Symptoms such as dizziness, weakness and tummy ache precede a gradual loss of consciousness, during which a sensation of floating or fading may be experienced, sometimes with loss of vision. The child who faints typically slumps to the ground and appears pale and lifeless. The period of unconsciousness is very brief and usually lasts less than sixty seconds; it is due to a sudden drop in blood pressure and heart rate which causes a reduction in the amount of blood and oxygen getting to the brain. While recovery is rapid, pallor and a feeling of tiredness may persist.

During the attack, the child should be placed in the recovery position, i.e on her side, until she regains consciousness. Don't try to revive the child by giving mouth-to-mouth resuscitation or by lifting her up, as this can aggravate the already poor supply of blood and oxygen to the brain and may cause a convulsion with stiffening and arching of the body and jerking of the limbs, which could be mistaken for an epileptic convulsion. The convulsive phase following a faint is usually very brief and is essentially a protective mechanism whereby the body tries to pump blood back to the brain.

Fainting seizures do not cause any form of brain damage. Simple fainting attacks are more common in adolescent girls. In children, recurrent fainting episodes appear to be due to an immaturity of the developing autonomic nervous system that controls heart rate and blood pressure. Factors that may trigger this type of seizure include pain, fear, fasting or a warm, stuffy environment. Fainting episodes can usually be prevented in the older child by avoiding potential triggering factors, and sitting or preferably lying down when feelings of dizziness or weakness develop.

Blue breath-holding spells

Breath-holding spells are common in toddlers, particularly between the ages of fifteen months and two and a half years. The typical child is often overactive, walks at an early age and has a tendency to temper-tantrums. The spell begins with the child becoming upset, either because she is not having her way or she has been chastised. A cry, sometimes unusually harsh, is followed by breath-holding, cyanosis (blue colour) of the lips and face, loss of consciousness, with stiffening and arching backward of the neck and body, followed by limpness. The stiffening phase usually lasts for fifteen to thirty seconds, and occasionally some jerking of the arms and legs may occur, which makes parents worry about the possibility of epilepsy. Once an attack occurs, it is best to put the child lying on her side and wait until the episode is over. Breath-holding spells can be a very frightening experience for parents, particularly during the limpness phase when they often feel that their child is lifeless or has died. Fortunately, recovery is rapid — within a minute. But the child may be drowsy or irritable for a short time afterwards.

Breath-holding spells are not serious and will not cause brain damage. Children prone to these episodes will grow out of them by the age of three and a half.

No specific treatment is required. Parents are advised to try to anticipate episodes and to avoid situations that might trigger an attack. This can sometimes be achieved by quickly removing or diverting the child from a potentially provocative situation. Some children can learn to self-induce breath-holding episodes in order to get their way and gain attention. This often happens where attacks initially occur frequently and the child learns to enjoy the fuss that is created, and the attention that is focussed on her.

White breath-holding spells

White breath-holding spells are similar to blue spells, and indeed may overlap in the same child. White breath-holding spells are also called reflex-anoxic seizures. The episode typically follows a minor traumatic event such as a bump to the head. On impact, the child suddenly collapses, and becomes very pale and limp. It is quite similar to a faint and indeed the mechanism is the same, with a sudden fall in blood pressure and heart rate following the shock of the impact. This type of episode after a trivial blow to the head can be particularly distressing for parents because it appears that the impact has been severe enough to cause the loss of consciousness, which is not the case. Fortunately, these episodes last only about sixty seconds and are followed by a quick recovery. If the child is picked up suddenly during the attack in an attempt to resuscitate her, she may go rigid, or her limbs may start jerking. The best thing is to put the child in the recovery position, lying down, until consciousness returns. Just like fainting seizures and blue breath-holding attacks, white breath-holding spells do not cause any brain damage. These episodes usually occur in toddlers and most children outgrow them by the age of four or five years.

Self-induced unconsciousness

School children sometimes practise this trick to get out of class. By taking several deep breaths in the squatting position and then standing up, blowing hard and at the same time closing the nostrils with the fingers, a sudden loss of consciousness occurs. The mechanism is similar to breath-holding. Alternatively, a friend can help bring on the attack by suddenly compressing the chest from behind after the deep breaths are taken. This is a harmless trick but it can cause concern for teachers or parents, particularly if the child does not admit to bringing on the attack herself. Rapid over-breathing or hyperventilating can also induce loss of consciousness, and outbreaks of this hysterical phenomenon have been reported in schools.

Ritualistic spells

Young children between the ages of eighteen months and three years often engage in ritualistic seizure-like behaviour when they are tired, particularly before they go off to sleep at night, but also when they are tired or bored during the day. This ritualistic activity usually consists of slow, rhythmic twisting movements of the arms and legs, and sometimes facial grimacing accompanied by blank staring. The child may appear unresponsive, but usually they alert immediately to either calling their name or lifting and cuddling them. Ritualistic behaviour of this type is harmless, and the child will grow out of it. It would appear that such children find the movements stimulating and relaxing, so it is probably better to allow them continue without interruption.

Staring spells and day-dreaming

Day-dreaming is common in children. Many switch off if they are tired or bored, particularly in the classroom. Often the main concern is the possibility that the child is suffering from 'absence' or 'petit mal' epilepsy (see p123). In my experience, when day-dreaming occurs exclusively in the classroom it is most likely not due to epilepsy but rather to boredom, tiredness or inability to keep up with the schoolwork. In the typical day-dream or switching-off episode, the child is found staring into space and will usually respond to calling their name or tapping the side of the face. In contrast, the child having an absence seizure suddenly ceases all activity, is unresponsive to any form of stimulation, stares blankly, often with fluttering of the eyelids, and has a characteristic vacant look. Absence seizures occur more commonly towards the end of the day, when they are observed by the parents. When staring spells or day-dreaming are a regular occurrence in class, then consideration should be given to overtiredness, boredom or inability to keep up with the schoolwork. In the latter situation an educational assessment by a psychologist may be needed.

'Alice in Wonderland' spells

Children in the six to ten age group, particularly girls, sometimes complain about seeing objects or people as either very small (micropsia) or very large (macropsia), or even changing in size. When this symptom occurs in isolation it does not appear to cause any distress for the child. The complaint may last for minutes, and frequently recurs. These can also occur in migraine and in some forms of epilepsy, but with these conditions there are always other symptoms. Parents can be assured that the 'Alice in Wonderland' spell is not harmful, and that the child will grow out of it. It appears to be caused by the developing visual system in the brain. It is said that Lewis Carroll based the fairy tale on his own personal experiences of this phenomenon.

Febrile seizures

Seizures and convulsions triggered by high temperature occur in up to 5 per cent of children between the ages of six months and five years. Febrile seizures often result in loss of consciousness, with stiffening of the body and jerking or twitching of the limbs. The duration of the seizure is usually only minutes, but can be much longer. Once the seizure is over, the child usually recovers consciousness rapidly.

Febrile seizures can occur with a variety of infections, but the most common cause is a viral infection of the throat, such as tonsillitis. Seizures tend to recur, but this tendency gradually diminishes as the child gets older, and by the age of four or five years the problem resolves. There is often a family history of similar seizures. Febrile convulsions are not a form of epilepsy.

Treatment involves lowering the temperature by removing clothing, tepid sponging, and using a fan if available, in addition to giving paracetamol. Aspirin and medications containing aspirin should not be given to children with fever because of the danger of causing acute liver damage. If fever persists despite this approach, the child should be examined by the family doctor because an antibiotic may be required. Treatment with daily medication, as in epilepsy, is not needed, but the child may be prescribed a tranquilliser in the form of suppositories that can be given at the start of a convulsion to stop it. Febrile seizures are not serious and can usually be managed by parents at home.

Useful address

The Irish Epilepsy Association, 249 Crumlin Road, Dublin 12. Tel. (01) 4554133.

Dr Joe McMenamin MD, FRCPI, FRCPC (PAED), FRCPC (NEUR) is a Consultant Paediatric Neurologist at Our Lady's Hospital for Sick Children, Crumlin, and Beaumont Hospital, Dublin.

GROWTH AND DEVELOPMENT

PROFESSOR HILARY HOEY

We are all fascinated by how our children grow and develop, and we can't help comparing them with other children of the same age. A child's progress can be viewed from two angles: physical growth, which is mainly height and weight, and developmental growth, which is the process by which he acquires new skills, such as sitting up, walking and talking.

In this chapter, consultant paediatrician Professor Hilary Hoey describes normal growth and the developmental milestones in infancy and childhood.

NORMAL GROWTH

To grow well a child needs good health, good nutrition and a loving home. The first stage of growth occurs in the womb before the child is born, and depends on many factors, including parents' height, the health of the mother, and good antenatal care. Smoking causes poor growth of the baby.

Height

From birth to two years the child grows very rapidly. Height is inherited, and is related to both parents' heights. The baby's size at birth and in the first two years of life is related more to the mother's build than the father's, but from two years onwards the father has a more marked influence. It is therefore not possible to predict future adult height until after the age of two.

The average healthy child will grow to be approximately twice as tall as he is on his second birthday. After the age of two, the growth rate slows down to 4–6cm ($1\frac{1}{2}$–2in) per year, until puberty, when there is an adolescent growth spurt. A girl has her adolescent growth spurt early in puberty, about the age of ten, and her growth is almost complete by the time she has had her first period. After this, she only grows approximately 5cm (2in) over the next two years.

Boys, on the other hand, start puberty approximately one year later than girls, at about the age of eleven, and do not have their growth spurt until the end of adolescence, after they have developed pubic hair, enlargement of their genitalia (sexual organs), facial hair and deepening of the voice, all of which take approximately two years.

The timing of puberty is very variable. In Ireland, the average age at which a girl gets her first period is 13.5 years. This is related to the family pattern — the age at which her mother had her first period. It may be delayed if the child is unwell. Many children are small in early childhood, but continue to grow for a longer period, thus gaining extra centimetres; they have a late adolescent growth spurt, resulting in a good adult height, similar to those who were tall, had an early puberty and stopped growing sooner.

Late puberty is the most common cause of short stature in childhood, and is called constitutional growth delay. Usually one or both parents have also had a late puberty, and these children need no treatment other than reassurance.

The most important aspect of a child's growth is the rate at which he is growing. If he is small but growing at a normal rate, he is normal. However, if he is small but growing at a poor rate, he is abnormal. You and your doctor can monitor his rate of growth.

A child should be treated according to his age and not his size. Tall children have been shown to mature faster, as they are given more responsibility, whereas small children tend to mature more slowly, as they are treated as being less able.

Weight

Weight is a more variable measurement than height, as it is influenced by many factors, such as what the child has eaten and if any recent infection, such as a cold, has affected the child's appetite. The average weight at birth is 3.5kg (7.5lb). In the first four days the baby loses weight, but he regains his birth weight by ten days. He doubles his birth weight by four to six months, trebles it by one year, quadruples it by two years, and then very slowly continues to gain weight until adolescence. A child who is below average weight may well be very healthy. However, he should be monitored by a doctor to see if he is gaining weight at a satisfactory rate.

Head size

A child's head size and shape is often similar to his parents'. At birth, there is a gap between the bones on the top of the head (the anterior fontanelle), and this is why the top of a baby's skull feels soft. The gap gradually closes between twelve and eighteen months of age. Many babies also have a gap at the back of their heads (the posterior fontanelle), which closes after about two months. A child's head may become flattened on one side if he always lies on the same side, or he may be born with an asymmetrical (misproportioned) head. This usually rights itself and these children develop normally.

NORMAL DEVELOPMENT

Each child develops skills and personality at his own pace. Children may be advanced in one skill and relatively retarded in another; for example, they may be advanced in walking and slow in speech. These characteristics run in families and often there is no reason. This is usually unrelated to their future intelligence.

The rate of development depends on the growing maturation of the child's nervous system, which is largely influenced by his inherited pattern. Stimulation, however, and delight by parents at a child's progress, provide a very good incentive to develop, and it has been shown that children who are unloved do not develop well, either physically or mentally. Pre-term (premature) babies are later in their developmental milestones, as they have been born early and have missed time in the womb.

DEVELOPMENTAL MILESTONES

Birth to three months

The primitive reflexes are present from birth, and allow for an involuntary response to a stimulus, for example, when you put your finger into a baby's palm, his hand closes on it; when you hold him in the standing position and his foot touches a surface, he walks.

The average baby smiles at approximately six weeks of age. He then starts to coo, gurgle, and squirm when tickled. At six weeks he is alert when awake, follows with his eyes, and stares at people and objects. At three months he will hold a rattle if placed in his hand, but cannot pick it up himself. At this age he may also turn his head in response to sound.

Six months

He will sit with support and may sit unsupported for a few seconds. He will also bear weight on his legs and bounce with delight when held. He can now reach for objects, pick them up with the palm of his hand, and put them to his mouth.

Nine months

At this age he may crawl (some children do not go through the crawling stage).   He can use a thumb and finger to grip, and is therefore able to pick up small objects. He also starts to 'make strange' with people.

Twelve months

He can now pull himself to standing position and walk around the furniture. He can say a few words with meaning, for example 'Dada', 'teddy'. He also enjoys games like 'Peek-aboo'.

Eighteen months

He will now walk without support, usually unsteadily and with feet apart. He can put three cubes on top of each other, scribble with a pencil, and feed himself. He will understand simple commands and will fetch objects. He shows a desire for attention. A period of negativism usually begins, where he wishes to do the opposite of what he is asked.

Two years

He walks more steadily, runs, and can kick a ball. He can turn handles, unscrew jars, and put on some clothes, such as a sock or cardigan. He puts two to three words together and may be potty-trained.

Three years

He walks steadily and rides a tricycle. He becomes less negative and is anxious to please. He plays with other children, starts to count, loves stories, can say sentences and asks questions. He becomes aware of and is interested in his genitalia (sexual organs).

Four years

He can now skip and stand on one leg. He can also dress and undress. He boasts and is very imaginative, telling unlikely stories to explain his misbehaviour. He has no idea of truth or untruth. Children use both hands equally up to the age of three to four years, and then show a preference for one.

All these timings are based on statistics, but most children will learn these skills sooner or later than the average child. If your child is later than average in one or two skills, such as walking or talking, this is not usually a sign that he is backward or low in intelligence; nor does very rapid development suggest a very high intelligence. A mentally backward child is usually late in all fields except, occasionally, sitting and walking. The early indications of normal development are that when the child is awake he is alert and interested, smiling at six weeks, and following with his eyes at three months. However, some slow starters make a great spurt forward later on.

Numerous factors affect the age at which various skills are learned. If your child is markedly late in acquiring a skill, this should be discussed with your doctor. If he is late in talking, he should have his hearing checked. Delayed speech may be related to his family pattern or to lack of people talking to him, but it may also be related to a hearing loss.

The important thing is to have your child's rate of development checked regularly by your family doctor or clinic doctor. This is recommended at six weeks, six to eight months, eighteen months, two and a half years, and at school entry. Half-yearly height and weight measurements can be done at home, and any worries discussed with your doctor. A baby-book or notebook recording your child's measurements and milestones may be both fun to do and provide useful information should problems develop later on.

Hilary Hoey MA, MD, FRCPI, DCH is Professor of Paediatrics at Trinity College, Dublin, and a Consultant Paediatrician at the National Children's Hospital, Harcourt Street, Dublin, and Our Lady's Hospital for Sick Children, Crumlin, Dublin.

HOW CHILDREN UNDERSTAND ILLNESS

PROFESSOR CIARAN O'BOYLE

Any illness in a child is a cause for concern, especially if the child is hospitalised, even for a short period. In the midst of their own anxiety, parents can easily forget that the child too may be anxious, and often suffering from unnecessary fears that she cannot even express.

A child's understanding of the nature, causes and treatment of illness is very different from that of an adult, and psychologist Professor Ciaran O'Boyle explains how a child's views can change as her thinking develops from infancy to adolescence. If we understand how children perceive their illness, we can communicate better with them and reduce their anxieties, which in turn will help them get better sooner.

CHILDREN AND ILLNESS

Many illnesses in childhood are mild and are experienced as a brief period of relative inactivity, concentrated concern by parents, and spoiling, in the midst of otherwise busy lives. Often, parents cope with their children's illnesses without any professional help or with just one or two visits to the family doctor. Many serious diseases such as rheumatic fever and tuberculosis have almost disappeared, while others that in the past required years of bed-rest in hospital, can now be cured quickly by means of an operation. However, advances in medicine and surgery sometimes make emotional demands on children and their parents such as were not foreseen even ten years ago. Illnesses such as leukaemia, which previously were fatal, can often be cured, and the harmful effects of diseases such as cystic fibrosis can be reduced, but families may face years of uncertainty about their child's future and be forced to witness them undergoing arduous medical treatment. Such chronic conditions require significant psychological adjustment by the child and her family.

A child with a chronic illness may have to face unpleasant and often painful symptoms, as well as having to cope with treatment procedures that may also be painful. Drugs may have unpleasant side-effects, such as loss of hair or other changes in appearance. Treatment may mean many trips to hospital, which can result in separation from the family and disruption of school attendance, learning and friendships.

Because human beings seek meaning in their lives, sick children require explanations for their conditions and their treatment. Great anxiety and distress can be caused by the child misunderstanding something important about her condition, and the parent, doctor or nurse who is not aware of how children think is unlikely to be able to get to the root of the problem. It is not until about eleven to twelve years of age that a child is capable of fully understanding illness as a complex process involving many factors.

HOW CHILDREN THINK

In order to understand how children perceive illness, it is necessary to understand the way in which children's thinking develops at different stages of their lives. The stages of thought development can be categorised broadly as follows:

Infants and toddlers

Babies are born with a few simple reflexes, such as grasping and sucking. The newborn baby can distinguish human voices from other sounds, and prefers to listen to its mother's voice and to heartbeats. While they cannot yet focus their eyes, they can see, and prefer to look at complex patterns, and at patterns that resemble faces. As the infant develops and begins to explore the world, she acquires a range of physical and mental abilities. At first, objects only exist for the baby when they can be seen. If you hide a toy with which a five-month-old is playing, she will not search for it. However, if you do this with a twelve-month-old, the baby will search for the toy. This is because babies learn at about seven to twelve months that objects are permanent, that they exist even when they cannot be seen. The infant's memory is developing at this stage, and she can now remember that there was an object in the first place.

This development has important implications for the manner in which we deal with young children when they are ill. By their third or fourth month, infants show that they recognise and prefer certain people — by smiling and cooing more when they see these familiar faces or hear their voices, although they are still fairly receptive to strangers. At about seven or eight months, however, this indiscriminate acceptance changes, and many children begin to 'make strange'. Parents are often upset to find that their previously friendly infant starts to cry at the approach of a stranger. At about the same time, most infants begin to show distress over being separated from their parents, especially the mother. This is known as separation anxiety, which peaks at about fourteen to eighteen months, and then gradually declines. By the time they are about three years old, most children are secure enough in their parents' absence to interact comfortably with other children and adults.

Separation and stranger anxiety are important elements in a child's development because they ensure that children develop a secure attachment to a safe adult, usually the parent, and avoid potentially unsafe contacts with strangers. The timing of these fears coincides with the growth of the child's mental abilities, especially memory. From about six months, infants get better at remembering past events and comparing things that happened in the past with what is happening now. This makes it possible for the baby to detect and sometimes to fear unusual or unpredictable events or people. The child is also better able to recall the earlier presence of an object or person that has disappeared from view. The infant cannot 'miss' its mother unless it can recall her presence a moment ago and compare this with her absence now. When the parent leaves the room, the infant is aware that something is wrong, and this can lead to distress. The seven-month-old now knows that her mother exists even when she cannot be seen, and is therefore more likely to be upset when left alone or in a strange place. When the child can remember past instances of separation and return, she becomes better able to anticipate the return of the absent parent, and the anxiety diminishes.

Because of the damaging effects of separation and stranger anxiety, children's hospitals now provide more facilities for parents to remain with their sick children and to be involved in their nursing. The need for the parents' presence decreases after about four years of age, when separation and stranger anxiety decrease significantly.

Because of the very limited mental abilities of toddlers, it is better to explain things to them visually, for example, if the child's leg is to be put in plaster, then why not bandage the leg of a favourite teddy or doll, so that she understands what this means. Toddlers have little understanding of time, and past and present mean nothing to them. Telling your hospitalised three-year-old that you will be back in the afternoon will mean little to her. Telling her that you will be back after she has had a sleep would be better, and leaving a glove, handbag or coat will provide tangible evidence that you will return.

From three to seven years

A four-year-old falls off his bicycle and announces, 'I fell off because it was Ciara's birthday'. While it seems obvious to us that the birthday did not cause the accident, the child appears to think it did. Three years later, however, the same child will say 'I fell off my bicycle because the front wheel skidded and I went over the top'. He has now acquired sophisticated notions about cause and effect.

During these years, the child learns a great deal about the world and begins to use symbols such as language and concepts. Thinking continues to develop, but it is still very limited in that children of this age can only deal with one aspect of a situation at a time: they cannot relate what they learn from one experience to another similar one; they do not distinguish clearly between fantasy and reality. Their thinking is dominated by what they see or experience. The child relies totally on her own view of things and finds it impossible to look at things from another person's point of view. A four-year-old, for example, will inform her teacher that her sister has no sister. Children of this age attribute life to objects. One four-year-old told his teacher that the moon was alive. When asked why, he answered, 'because we are'.

At this stage children define health as a state that enables them to do things, such as going outside or playing with their friends. Health in other people is judged by external concrete signs such as rosy cheeks, clear eyes and nice skin. Illness is defined in terms of a single external symptom that is usually observed in connection with the illness. The child attributes the source of the illness to be either a person or object that is near to but not necessarily touching the ill person, or to an event or activity that occurs before the onset of the illness. The child does not understand the idea of cause and effect.

This is illustrated in the following conversations with children at this age:

'What are measles?'
'Measles are bumps on your arm.'
'How do people get measles?'
'From other people.'
'How do people get measles from other people?'
'When you walk near them.'
'How does walking near them give you measles?'
'When you go near them.'

'What is a cold?'
'It's coughing a lot.'
'How do people get colds?'
'From other children.'
'How do other children give you a cold?'
'You catch it, that's all.'

These children concentrate on a single concrete aspect of the illness, bumps for measles and coughing for a cold, and believe that simply being near someone is sufficient to cause the illness.

The importance of understanding the child's point of view can be seen even in something as simple as using a stethoscope. Doctors often respond to children's fear of the stethoscope by warming it, assuming that the cold metal against the child's skin is what causes the negative response. However, when four and five-year-olds were asked about the stethoscope, they made no mention of coldness, but told researchers that the purpose of the stethoscope was to discover 'if I have a heart'. As the child sees it, if the doctor doesn't find a heart, then they could die.

Illness as punishment

Children do not distinguish clearly between the real world and their fantasy world. Any adult who has had to play with a child's invisible playmate knows this. Children in plaster often think that once the cast is removed, they will at once, as if by magic, be completely well. If unprepared for the reality that faces them, they may express their anger and disappointment in behaviour such as demands for attention, bedwetting and even soiling.

From three to seven years, children's ideas regarding illness frequently involve punishment, guilt and self-blame. In one study, 90 per cent of children in hospital with heart problems and diabetes answered the question, 'Why do children get sick?' with 'Because they are bad'. Hospitalised children often ascribe the cause of their illness to disobeying their parents, and interpret their hospitalisation as punishment.

Mark, a little boy of six, was admitted to hospital with infectious osteomyelitis, a painful infection of the bone marrow which affected his thigh and the bones of his face. After some time he became increasingly upset, refused to eat and began to vomit for no apparent reason. Eventually, a psychologist was brought to see him. When he was asked, 'What is the matter with your face; why is it all swollen?', he replied in matter-of-fact tones, 'It's because I bite my nails'. His distress was caused by his blaming himself for his condition because, as he saw it, he had done something naughty. His parents confirmed that he was a nail-biter, and that they had often told him it was a dirty habit. They also recalled the doctor saying that perhaps the infection had been caused by dirt getting into his mouth. Mark himself had made the connection and blamed himself for his condition.

Children in the three to seven age-group define something as wrong if it merits punishment. Their logic goes: what is bad is punished, therefore what is punished is bad. Since the young child does not understand that things can happen by chance or accident, she seeks a reason for everything. Therefore, when suffering from illness or pain, she often automatically assumes that it is punishment, and searches for the naughty behaviour that must account for the punishment. Such thinking is also common when a family member dies, and the child mistakenly believes that something she did was responsible. A further example of this thinking is: 'If bad follows bad and good follows good, how can bad-tasting medicine or painful injections make you better?' It is important to understand this type of thinking in children, because it leads to guilt and anxiety, and can result in depression.

From seven to twelve years

The major change in children's thinking at about seven or eight years is that the child can now focus on more than one aspect of a situation at the same time. The child also begins to think logically and can look at a situation from someone else's point of view, but still does not differentiate the mind from the body. Health is defined in more abstract terms. The child can describe health in terms of feeling good, feeling like doing things, being happy, and so forth. She begins to understand that illnesses can result in a number of symptoms, some of which are less obvious than others. Children also begin to understand more clearly that there is a direct link between the source of a disease and the disease itself. However, illness can still be interpreted as punishment: just as contact with dirt or germs causes illness, so does bold behaviour, as illustrated in the following exchange with a seven-year-old:

'What is cancer?'
'Cancer is when you're very sick and you go to the hospital and you throw up a lot, and stuff.'
'How do people get cancer?'
'From smoking without their mother's permission.'
'How does this give you cancer?'
'You shouldn't do that — it's bad.'

Reverting to childish behaviour

Illness generally involves going to bed and being looked after. When we are ill, we like to be cared for and we often revert to a stage of dependency on others. Most of us readily permit ourselves this agreeable experience, which can act as a sort of reward for being ill and out of circulation. Some young children, when ill, lapse back into a state of helpless infancy, and during convalescence may have to re-learn many of their social skills. Parents should not be surprised to see older children, even adolescents, reverting to more 'childish behaviour' and becoming more demanding when they are ill.

Some children, however, do not show this type of regression when ill. Nature appears to have given children a powerful driving force which pushes their psychological and physical development forward. All children enjoy practising newly acquired abilities — try stopping a toddler who has just discovered climbing, and you will get the idea. Young children who have struggled to master independent eating, washing and toileting, do not give up these achievements easily when they become ill. Restriction of movement, for example in a toddler with a broken leg, can be even more upsetting than the illness itself. Many of us have seen young toddlers who have only just learned to walk, stand up stubbornly in their cots for the whole course of an illness such as measles.

ADOLESCENCE

At about eleven or twelve years of age, the child's thinking is more like that of an adult. Adolescents think more abstractly and have a more mature understanding of illness. The child is now influenced more by what he or she knows, than by what is seen. The role of friends and peers becomes more important. This can lead to problems, especially when there are things that everyone else is doing but which the adolescent cannot do because of illness or disease. Physical handicaps or deformities can become very difficult to deal with at this age because appearance is so important to the adolescent. Since adolescents have the capacity to think abstractly, they can now compare themselves with an ideal self or body image, and such comparisons can lead to distress.

HOW CHILDREN PERCEIVE PAIN

The belief that illness results from misbehaving is common in children and has important implications for dealing with children in pain. For example, children with burns who blame themselves for their condition may complain less about their pain. Since doctors and nurses assess the degree of pain on the basis of complaint, the level of pain being experienced by such children is likely to be underestimated. In an interesting research study, psychologists at University College Cork looked at children's understanding of what caused pain. They studied 680 Irish schoolchildren between the ages of five and fourteen years. Up to about seven years of age, pain was described as something that is concrete, limited to certain parts of the body, dominated by what it feels like, and there was little or no understanding of the link between pain and illness, nor of the value of pain as a warning system.

After about seven, thinking becomes more abstract. Pain can be anywhere and 'can be inside you'. Descriptions are more vivid and the child begins to understand that pain has a psychological component: 'pain is something that hurts you...feels like knives and forks stabbing into you...you feel miserable and unhappy and you start crying'.

At about eleven or twelve, the child can think in purely abstract terms. Whereas the younger child generally has a passive view of pain, the older child sees pain as something that has to be coped with or borne, and she now knows that there is such a thing as mental pain, which may be more difficult to cure.

HOW CHILDREN PERCEIVE DEATH

Children's understanding of death is broadly in line with their understanding of illness. Under the age of four or five, they generally ignore the phenomenon or else respond with puzzled or somewhat callous interest. Between five and eight they become very interested in death, associate it with aggressive feelings and fears, regard it as a punishment for misdeeds, but also as reversible. Young children often distinguish between 'being dead' and 'being dead for ever'. Death is not recognised as accidental: it always happens for a reason, usually a retaliation for some wrongdoing, often as a result of the child's own bad wishes. It is not until about nine years old that they acquire a rational understanding of death. When children experience a death in the family, they may respond by becoming good and conscientious, as if this will revive the dead person. This type of bargaining behaviour is sometimes seen in adults who are bereaved.

When a family member dies, children may suffer anxiety and guilt. Adults often deal with children in such circumstances by trying to protect them from what is happening. They may be shunted off to a relative until after the funeral. There is often great reluctance to let children see a dead body. Explanations are usually given in the form 'Granny has gone to sleep' or 'God wanted another angel'. Parents must use their own judgement, but in general, truthful, realistic explanations are best, and children should be included in arrangements. Not to do so creates a situation in which the child's imagination can take over, and parents may not be aware of the unnecessary distress the child may be suffering as a result of being excluded.

UNDERSTANDING YOUR CHILD'S POINT OF VIEW

Communicating with a sick child is quite different from communicating with a sick adult. Children can be devastatingly frank, but can just as easily be totally confused by what they see and hear. Young children often cannot explain what is wrong, and cannot identify pain, and may come to surprising conclusions about the treatment they receive. Adults' explanations to children regarding illness often assume that the child has a more developed understanding of the world than is actually the case. Until the age of nine or ten, for example, a child cannot be expected to appreciate that a number of different symptoms may be associated with a single illness, or understand the progression of illness through different phases, or to understand the logic of taking medicine by mouth for a skin rash.

Babies, even when ill, need sensory stimulation. Providing toys dangling before their eyes, propping them up to get a view of the world, talking to and playing with them when their condition allows, and encouraging interaction with older children, all help to reduce their feelings of deprivation.

Before the age of about eleven, children find it difficult to understand explanations about internal bodily processes and conditions that affect them, such as haemophilia or epilepsy. In general, explanations to younger children should be as concrete as possible, preferably making use of drawing, stories and play. This is especially relevant when dealing with pain. The non-verbal behaviour used by younger children in role-playing, miming or doll's play can highlight aspects of pain that they are unable to describe. Drawing can also be particularly useful here. When preparing children for operations or tests, the emphasis should be placed on what they will see and observe (lights in the operating room, nurse's uniforms), and if possible they should be given some of the equipment to examine and play with. A teddybear or favourite doll going through the same procedure as themselves can be an invaluable aid.

The belief that illness results from misbehaving is common in children. Consequently, they may interpret uncomfortable or painful diagnostic and treatment procedures as punishment. Serious illness, handicap or the death of a child is a major stress not only for parents but for the child's brothers and sisters. They are likely, especially if under the age of seven or eight, to feel guilt, as if their past normal rivalry with the sick child had caused the misfortune. In addition, the parents may be so preoccupied with the child who is ill that the psychological needs of the other children are not met.

Children generally rely on adults to help them make sense of their illness. When parents and doctors are themselves so worried and preoccupied that they cannot listen to the child's fears and provide truthful and rational explanations that the child can understand, then the child is likely to be upset. We must not ignore children's concerns when they are ill. Parents and medical personnel often talk about children in their presence, as if they were not there. This upsets children. As John, aged five, put it, 'The doctors looked at my throat, at my tummy, and at my ears, but they didn't look at ME'.

Professor C A O'Boyle BSc, PhD, Reg Psychol (APsSI), CPsychol (AFBPsS) is Professor of Psychology at the Medical School of the Royal College of Surgeons in Ireland. He is also qualified as a pharmacologist and has a particular interest in the areas of stress and pain.

HYPERACTIVITY

DR PAUL CARSON

'He fidgets, he's restless, he can't concentrate on anything.'

'He's bright, but he's doing badly at school.'

'He disrupts the whole family.'

'We never get a full night's sleep with him'

'He has us driven up the walls!'

These are the sort of typical remarks that parents of hyperactive children make. However, as general practitioner Dr Paul Carson explains, there are many other reasons why a child may be constantly overactive and behave in an anti-social manner, and these should all be considered before a child is labelled as truly hyperactive.

THE HYPERACTIVE CHILD

It is important to appreciate that there is a wide range of 'normal' behaviour in children. An exuberant and active child who plays and lives to the full should not be confused with the disorganised and disruptive child whose activities show no set pattern. The normal but energetic child will be happy and interested in playtime, whereas the hyperactive child loses interest quickly and moves from one activity to another almost at random. He never truly seems at peace with himself or his friends.

About two thirds of all hyperactive children are boys. The hyperactive child often has fair skin, blue eyes and blond or red hair. He may be left-handed, have a finicky appetite and a pronounced thirst. There are, of course, exceptions to these general traits.

HOW TO RECOGNISE THE HYPERACTIVE CHILD

Inattentiveness: he is unable to remain attentive to any one subject or game; he will lose interest quickly and switch his attention to some other activity in minutes. He seems unable to listen, even to a story, without his attention wandering constantly. He engages in disorganised, restless, ceaseless activity, fidgets all the time, is always 'on the go', but rarely does anything constructive. This restless behaviour is noticeable day and night, and the child is often a poor, fitful sleeper.

Behavioural problems: he is very disruptive; he disturbs and distracts children at games, at school, or during any form of organised activity. He frequently speaks out of turn, and usually in the middle of someone else's conversation. He often makes irritating, repetitive noises, such as humming, clicking of fingers and so on. He is aggressive and belligerent, and is often involved in minor fights at school. He is very disobedient and responds poorly to reprimands.

Learning problems: it is reckoned that as many as 50 per cent of these children have definite learning problems and noticeably lag behind their peers in academic performance. The child may have difficulty retaining spoken words or distinguishing individual written words. He may find it difficult to pronounce letters. His spelling is likely to be poor. He can add and subtract on his fingers, but poorly on paper. He may have problems grasping and applying new information. He may be dyslexic and may reverse individual letters when writing.

Immaturity: the hyperactive child lags behind his peers in his psychological and emotional development. This is reflected in his choice of younger friends, his interests, and his inability to cope with certain situations. He cries easily and is easily frightened. By the time they reach their teens, as many as 70 per cent of these children are still classified as immature.

Impulsiveness: without thinking of the consequences, the child will often dart from one place to the next. This can be life-threatening on a busy road.

Lack of friends: these children have great difficulty relating to children of their own age.

Low self-esteem: because of their behaviour and the effect it has on those around them, hyperactive children are difficult to love in any normal sense. They are unpopular with other children, which in turn reinforces their feelings of isolation.

Unhappy personality: parents often comment on how unhappy their disruptive child is.

SYMPTOM SCORE CARD

The following score card will help you assess your own child if you suspect hyperactivity. Most children will exhibit these features occasionally, or in certain circumstances (such as after a children's party where they have eaten a lot of sugary and highly coloured sweets). What distinguishes the truly hyperactive child is the 'constant' nature of their symptoms.

Score two points for each 'yes' answer	**Yes/No**
Restless, 'always on the go'?	_____
Fidgets almost all the time?	_____
Easily distracted?	_____
Easily frustrated?	_____
Demanding of time and attention?	_____
Short attention span?	_____
Disturbs other children constantly?	_____
Unpredictable behavioural pattern?	_____
Excitable, impulsive?	_____
Frequent, unpredictable, often inappropriate mood changes?	_____
Often has a glazed look in his eyes?	_____
More than usually thirsty?	_____

A score of six or less is normal. A score of six to twenty suggests your child's behaviour is bordering on the abnormal, and it would be worth your while having him assessed. A score of twenty or more reflects abnormal hyperactive behaviour, and your child should be assessed by a trained professional with an interest in this area. In addition, you should put him immediately on the special diet that is explained later in this chapter.

OTHER CONDITIONS THAT MAY CAUSE BEHAVIOUR PROBLEMS IN CHILDREN

There are many reasons why a child may have behaviour problems, and these should be ruled out before a diagnosis of hyperactivity can be made.

Asthma: unrecognised, poorly treated asthma often makes children moody and fractious. (See chapter on 'Respiratory Problems'.) Some asthma treatments, especially when used in combination, can make children 'high as kites'. The group of drugs known as bronchodilators (wheeze-relieving) can certainly produce this reaction. One group (called theophyllines) can cause depression and mood swings in susceptible children.

Eczema: this is an irritating, dry, itchy skin condition. (See chapter on 'Skin Conditions'.) If left untreated or badly treated, the sheer discomfort of it can result in irritable, bad tempered and difficult children. Parents are often at fault here. Because of a misguided fear of side-effects from the steroid medication often prescribed for eczema, they may decide not to use it as directed; they grossly undertreat, and the child is left to suffer (and scratch and be tormented, and in turn torment others).

Allergic rhinitis: this is probably one of the most unrecognised medical conditions affecting children. It is especially common among children with asthma and eczema, and may be mistakenly labelled as all-year-round 'hayfever'. It is in fact an allergic irritation of the lining of the nose and causes immense discomfort. Clues to look out for include: itchy, runny nose; constantly rubbing at the nose; constant sneezing; nasal blockage. The discomfort of this condition can only be appreciated by adults who suffer recurrent sinus problems.

Migraine: some children have frequent headaches with nausea, occasionally diet-related due to taking too much chocolate, cola or cheese. They resent interference, noise or physical activities. They can become moody and withdrawn.

Deafness: children can develop a condition called 'glue ear', in which fluid accumulates in the inner ear. This interferes with their hearing, sometimes dramatically and obviously, but occasionally moderately and not always easily recognised. Parents may feel the child is deliberately ignoring them, or teachers may mistake the child's lack of response as disobedience. A simple example will illustrate the point: the child is sitting in front of the TV with the volume up high, and in comes Dad who screams, 'turn that thing down!'. The partially deaf child doesn't hear the command and receives a clip around the ear for being heedless and disobedient. The child is stunned! He is punished for a command he hasn't heard and all protests are ignored. Multiply this by the number of times it can happen every day and you have a recipe for disaster.

Drug treatments: some children with long-standing medical conditions such as epilepsy or asthma may need to take medications every day. There is always a possibility that such treatments will cause behavioural problems, and it is worth airing these fears with your doctor if you suspect your child's mood has changed for the worse since starting or changing long-term medication.

Drug abuse: drug abuse, such as glue sniffing, under-age alcohol drinking, the use of 'crack', marijuana, heroin, etc is unfortunately becoming more and more common in our society. Children as young as nine years are becoming involved in the underground drug culture. Sudden changes in mood, becoming withdrawn, irritable, resentful, or displaying totally anti-social behaviour, are some of the features to look out for in this regard.

Sexual or physical abuse: mood and personality changes associated with sexual or physical abuse are many and varied. Even a fairly simple situation of bullying at school can psychologically scar a child and alter his mood for the worse. How much more so can the torment of constant sexual or physical abuse at home cause behavioural disturbances?

Because there are so many causes for mood and behaviour changes in children, your first port of call for help if you are having difficulty with your child's behaviour is your family doctor. He or she can physically examine the child to rule in or out the conditions listed above, or recommend psychological help where the problem is not true hyperactivity but rather some form of psychological difficulty.

TREATMENT FOR HYPERACTIVITY

You have now reached the decision point: your child shows all the features of hyperactivity; he has been assessed by your family doctor and possibly also by a clinical psychologist, and they agree that there are no physical or psychological factors causing this behaviour (or at least any that exist have been identified and are being dealt with). You are still left with a difficult-to-manage child. What can you do?

Diet restrictions

Certain foods and drinks, or more usually the chemicals contained within them, can cause or aggravate hyperactive behaviour. For this reason the following dietary restrictions should be applied rigidly.

- All foods and drinks containing certain additives must be avoided. An additive is a chemical added to a food or drink to colour, flavour or preserve. Hyperactive children seem to be unduly sensitive to these compounds, and become overstimulated. Additives are usually listed as E-numbers. This is a coding system to allow the manufacturers list their additives by number rather than by their rather long, complicated names.

  The E-numbers to avoid are: E102, E104, E110, E122, E123, E124, E127, E128, E129, E131, E132, E133, E142, E150, E151, E153, E154, E155, E161g, E173, E180, E210, E211, E212, E213, E214, E215, E216, E217, E218, E219, E220, E221, E222, E223, E224, E226, E227, E228, E230, E231, E232, E233, E234, E235, E249, E250, E251, E252, E310, E311, E312, E320, E321, E621, E622, E950, E951, E953, E965, E954, E966, E967.

  Because manufacturers may avoid using the E-number and choose to use the chemical name instead, it is a good idea to buy one of the many books available on this subject, which list the additives by both E-numbers, and chemical names (see Recommended Reading, p234).

- All flavourings, unless already clearly marked 'natural', must be avoided.

- Foods containing salicylates should also be avoided. Salicylates are compounds closely related to aspirin, and some hyperactive children are unduly sensitive to them. The salicylate foods are: dried fruits, berry fruits, oranges, apricots, pineapples, cucumbers, gherkins, tomato sauce, cola, endives, olives, grapes, almonds, liquorice, peppermints, honey, Worcester sauce.

- Salicylates are also found in medicines containing aspirin. Many over-the-counter medicines contain aspirin and should be avoided. If a pain-killer is required, then plain paracetamol may be used.

- In addition to foods/drinks containing any of the above substances, all medicinal syrups or tablets coloured red, green, orange, lemon or blue must be avoided. Also vitamin supplements, toothpastes, pastilles, lozenges, etc, if they contain these colours.

- If your child has a marked thirst as part of his symptoms, then a three-month trial of Evening Primrose Oil can be useful. Evening Primrose Oil is a fatty substance that occurs naturally in the human body, and the theory is that hyperactive children may not have enough (for a variety of reasons) and can benefit from supplementation. This may be obtained from your pharmacist or health food store.

You will quickly find this diet is NOT restrictive at all, in that good healthy foods are allowed and only packaged, highly processed and coloured/flavoured products banned.

Although parents often believe that their children are allergic to other foods, such as dairy products, this is rarely the case. Your family doctor can decide if extra tests are needed to identify offending foods.

Points to remember

- The symptoms may get worse at the start of the diet. Bear with this, as improvement usually shows after five days.

- After a few months some children are able to tolerate the salicylate-containing foods in reduced quantities (but not the additives).

- The diet has very little effect on a child with psychological or emotional problems.

- The diet should never be used as a punishment routine.

- The greatest problem lies with relations, neighbours, grandparents, etc who may think the whole idea of the diet quite absurd, and cheat behind the parents' back. If your child is away from you for any length of time and you cannot control what foods or sweets are likely to be offered, then pin a large badge onto his chest with the clear instructions: *'Do not give me sweets, crisps etc until you have asked my Mum!'*

- Hyperactivity is NOT all about diet. The diet is just one part of an overall programme of management, which will involve doctors, psychologists and family therapists. Occasionally a drug that stimulates the nervous system is used in some severe cases of hyperactivity, where all other approaches have failed.

GENERAL ADVICE

- Encourage homemade, wholesome meals and regular eating habits. Try to ensure that the child is hungry for food, so don't allow snacks between meals.

- See that he gets adequate rest, fresh air and exercise.

- Make sure the house is safe: if necessary, put perspex on vulnerable windows; do not leave valuable or dangerous objects around; place locks high up on doors.

- When you say 'no' you must mean it. Be consistent, and ensure cooperation with all the immediate and extended family. Try always to remain calm, speaking in a soft, controlled voice. Discourage excessive noise.

- If possible, ignore bad behaviour, or at least control your temper. On the other hand, reward good behaviour. More often than not, hyperactive children are ignored or pushed aside, leading to poor self-esteem. It is important to give praise when deserved.

- Try to arrange help. This must be someone who will respect the diet and programme. It is essential to have some time to yourself in order to maintain some semblance of normal life for your own sanity and self-esteem.

- If you have a choice, choose a school with small classes, as hyperactive children need a lot of individual attention.

- Encourage quiet moments. Put the child into a comfortable position, sitting or lying, with your arms around him. Encourage him to breathe deeply — in through the nose, allowing the abdomen to rise, and out through the mouth, allowing the abdomen to relax. This is particularly helpful after a tantrum, to restore equilibrium.

- Remember, more than anything else, your child's hyperactivity is something you have to *cope* with; it is not something for which you have to blame yourself. Involve your family doctor and any other professionals he/she may suggest. Good control is very much a team effort.

Useful address

Hyperactive Children's Support Group, 25 Lawnswood Park, Stillorgan, Co Dublin. (Please enclose 9" x 6" S.A.E., with 40p stamp, for reply.)

Dr Paul Carson BA, MB, BCh, BAO, DFPA is a GP in Dublin, where he runs an Asthma and Allergy Clinic for children. He is the author of a series of books on health problems in children, including one on the hyperactive child.

INFECTIOUS DISEASES

PROFESSOR DENIS GILL

In Ireland over the last one hundred years, many killer diseases such as smallpox have been virtually wiped out, while others such as polio have been eradicated. This is a direct result of public vaccination schemes. However, our children are still at risk from a large number of common infectious diseases. Many of these in their mild form will merely cause the child discomfort and irritability for a few days or weeks, but in severe cases they can have very damaging effects, and can even kill.

Vaccines are now widely available in Ireland for childhood infections such as measles, whooping cough and rubella (German measles), yet we still have a very low rate of immunisation. Consultant paediatrician Professor Denis Gill describes the most common infections and urges parents to avail of vaccination wherever possible.

Infectious diseases are an integral element in the daily life of many children and adults in the developing world. Whilst many of us in the West have to talk to our grandparents to learn of the ravages of polio and diphtheria, in the world's poorest countries up to one in five children will die before their first birthday, mostly because of infectious illnesses such as measles, whooping cough and tuberculosis. The appearance of the AIDS epidemic in the 1980s has taught the western world that infection remains a major cause of disease and death.

WHAT IS IMMUNISATION?

The words vaccination, immunisation and inoculation, though not strictly the same, can be used interchangeably for practical purposes. Immunisation is a method whereby a child is given a very dilute or weakened dose of a virus or bacterium, for example measles or mumps. The body responds as though it has been infected, and produces prolonged protection against that disease. Immunisation is, in a sense, a form of homoeopathy.

Immunisation can be presented in an oral solution, as with the polio vaccine, or as an injection, such as the MMR (measles, mumps, rubella) vaccine. Research is currently underway into the possibility of presenting the measles virus vaccine as a nasal spray, this being the route by which we naturally catch the illness. Measles immunisation may not provide life-long protection, as the natural illness does, but it will provide protection through childhood, and can be repeated. It is now recommended that the MMR vaccine be given in both the first and second decades of life.

WHY IMMUNISE?

Immunisation has probably been the single most beneficial health advance for children this century, and yet approximately 20 per cent of Irish children are not adequately immunised. The quality of vaccines is improving and the number of vaccines is increasing, so it is worth considering the following points:

- *Immunisation is safe.* Despite all the adverse media publicity, almost all children can receive vaccination and expect only minor reactions. Serious reactions are extremely rare. Most doctors never see them.

- *Immunisation works.* Some 95 to 100 per cent of children can expect protection following full immunisation.

- *Immunisation prevents disease.* Prevention is always better than treatment. Measles vaccine is preferable to measles infection.

- *Immunisation is extremely cost-effective.* It is much cheaper to prevent disease than to pay for its treatment and consequences.

WHY ARE SOME CHILDREN NOT IMMUNISED?

- *Some parents don't believe in immunisation.* Some groups of people remain unconvinced of the benefits of vaccination. Some religious groups see immunisation as interfering with nature.

- *Some parents think that natural disease gives better protection.* This may be so. But natural disease also causes death and suffering, things we could all do without, especially our children who depend on us to protect them.

- *Some parents are ignorant about, or indifferent to, the necessity of immunisation.* They may be disorganised and forget to have their children vaccinated.

- *Some doctors, nurses or other health professionals give misinformation.* There have been differing medical opinions and views about the side-effects of vaccines. Happily, Ireland, the US and WHO (World Health Organisation) now have clear guidelines on almost all of the issues involved in immunisation. In Ireland, information leaflets are available from the Department of Health (see Recommended Reading, p 234).

- *Some parents are afraid of side-effects, real or imagined.* No parent wishes to harm her child. The mental conflict involved in the decision to vaccinate can be very real. Reason says that immunisation is good for the child. On the other hand, emotion may argue that needles are painful, contain unknown substances, and could be harmful. News stories of vaccine-damaged children serve to accentuate these uncertainties and difficulties. If a child is damaged by a disease such as measles, polio or pertussis (whooping cough), this can be construed by some as the will of God. However, if a child suffers a vaccine reaction, some parents may feel guilty of inflicting this on the child. It is important to remember that severe vaccine reactions are very, very rare indeed.

- *Some believe that infectious diseases are no longer a threat.* Parents in developing countries see diseases such as polio and diphtheria maim and kill their children, but in Ireland we have to be reminded that these conditions still exist.

- *Parents wish to express their freedom to choose.* So long as only a small minority of parents express this opt-out wish, there should not be too many problems, but where there are large numbers of children who have not been immunised, infectious diseases will always be a danger.

WHEN TO IMMUNISE?

In Ireland, BCG is given at birth in most, but not all, Health Board areas. The three-in-one vaccine (DTP) is commenced at two to three months, and given as three injections over three months. The present vaccination programme is shown below. The schedules are not static, but are regularly reviewed and updated; for example, the HiB vaccine was added to the programme in 1992.

Immunisation programme

Birth	BCG (bacille calmette guerin — the tuberculosis vaccine)
2, 3, 4 months	DTP (diphtheria, tetanus, pertussis) + oral polio + HiB (Haemophilus influenzae B)
or	
2, 4, 6 months	DTP + oral polio + HiB
12-15 months	MMR (measles, mumps, rubella)
5 years	DTP + polio
10-14 years	MMR
	BCG (repeated if not immune)

WHAT INFECTIONS AND WHAT IMMUNISATIONS?

The very nature of childhood means being at risk from a myriad of illnesses, injuries and external events. The acquisition of immunity to illnesses and the attainment of maturity go hand in hand. The following are brief descriptions of some infectious illnesses and the vaccines that protect against them.

DIPHTHERIA

Diphtheria has always been a serious and very frightening disease. The diphtheria germ infects the throat and tonsils, and as a result, breathing is obstructed and becomes increasingly difficult. In fatal cases, the child slowly suffocates to death. The diphtheria germ also releases a toxin that can damage the heart.

The vaccine against diphtheria was developed in the 1940s and used widely from the 1950s onwards. It has been one of the most successful vaccines ever produced, resulting in the virtual eradication of diphtheria from the western world.

The diphtheria germ is still around. Cases are occasionally seen in the United States and in the UK (mainly among immigrants from the Indian sub-continents). An outbreak occurred in Russia in 1993 because of the disintegration of the immunisation service.

POLIOMYELITIS (Polio)

Poliomyelitis is a highly contagious virus, usually resulting in a flu-like illness, with fever, chills, malaise, aches and pains. In the past, when polio was a common illness, it was mostly indistinguishable from other viruses and resulted in complete recovery. However, about one in every thousand affected children got a serious dose. This could cause meningitis (inflammation of the lining of the brain), paralysis of the chest muscles, or paralysis of one or both legs. Paralysis of the chest muscles was treated by the infamous 'iron lungs' in which people had to spend months and sometimes years.

The polio virus vaccine, which is given by mouth as drops or a lump of sugar, gives superb protection. Paralytic polio has been all but wiped out by the vaccine. But people must not forget that the polio virus still survives, waiting to infect susceptible individuals.

PERTUSSIS (Whooping Cough)

Cause:	A common bacterium spread by infected patients, especially early in the illness.
Infectivity:	Highly contagious, particularly among people living in overcrowded housing.
Age-group:	Particularly affects infants in the first year or two of life.
Features:	The illness has three stages: a preparatory stage, a spasmodic coughing stage, and a convalescent stage. The whole illness may last from three weeks to three months. Some infants are seriously affected, others mildly so. Some 80 per cent of unvaccinated children will develop whooping cough. The most characteristic feature of pertussis is the whooping accompanied by cough. The distressing and prolonged cough may be

followed by episodes of blueness and vomiting. Affected infants become distressed and exhausted. They feed poorly, lose weight and sleep restlessly. They may have convulsions (fits).

Complications: Pneumonia, weight loss, prolonged cough, brain damage (from convulsions), encephalitis (inflammation of the brain), death (though this is now rare). The most frequent distressing feature of pertussis is the loss of sleep caused to parents and child, and the relative ineffectiveness of all medicines, including cough bottles, sedatives and antibiotics.

Severity rating: Moderate. Severe in infants under six months of age.

Vaccine: Effective. 80–90 per cent protection. Not recommended in the event of (a) major reaction to preceding dose, and (b) rare neurological disorders. Best discussed with your doctor.

MEASLES

Cause: A common virus.

Infectivity: Highly contagious. Tends to occur in epidemics.

Age-group: Any, but most likely in children from six months to three years.

Features: Measles is usually a miserable, self-limiting illness, with high temperature, rash, cough, sore eyes and loss of appetite. The affected child has red eyes, red skin, red throat, and often red ears. It is especially dangerous in children who are undernourished or whose resistance to infection is reduced.

Complications: Complications include ear infections, chest infections, convulsions, and on rare occasions inflammation of the brain. The rates of complications are high:

1 in 10 children with measles have complications.

1 in 100 children have to be hospitalised.

1 in 1000 children develops inflammation of the brain (encephalitis).

1 in 10,000 children dies.

1 in every 100,000 children will develop SSPE (sub acute sclerosing panencephalitis), a rare and devastating destruction of the brain, which results in dementia, gradual deterioration, and eventual death.

It is because of this complication rate that doctors in most countries of the world have voted in favour of the measles vaccine.

Immunity: Natural measles infection usually provides lifelong protection to the child. Measles in pregnancy is not thought to affect the foetus.

Severity rating: Worse in younger children and in those who are undernourished. Fatalities are rare in the developed world, but still common in the developing world, where it is estimated that two million children die each year as a result of measles.

Special precautions: Particularly dangerous in children suffering from leukaemia, or children on cortisone or similar drugs.

Vaccine: Highly effective. A weakened live virus. Given
                    by injection. May cause 'mini-measles', a very
                    mild form of measles.

MUMPS

Cause: A virus.

Infectivity: Highly contagious.

Age-group: Highest frequency in children of school age.

Features: Usually mild illness, with swelling of one or
                    both parotid (salivary) glands at the side of the
                    face. Associated with pain and loss of appetite.
                    Also fever, which lasts a few days. Usually
                    runs an uncomplicated course.

Complications: Meningoencephalitis (inflammation of the
                    brain); deafness, which may affect both ears
                    and be permanent; inflammation of the testicles
                    or ovaries, which can impair fertility. Mumps is
                    now thought to be one of the commonest
                    causes of permanent deafness in children.

Severity rating: Moderate. Deafness and sterility potentially
                    serious.

Vaccine: Live, weakened virus. Very effective. Injection
                    usually provides lifelong immunity.

VARICELLA (Chicken-pox)

Cause: A virus.

Infectivity: Highly contagious.

Age-group: Any, but usually pre-school.

Features: Blisters on the body, face and limbs. The
                    blisters crust after a few days. The rash is itchy.

The child may have a slight temperature, but is not usually very ill.

Complications: Infection of blisters. Rarely, pneumonia or encephalitis (inflammation of the brain).

Severity rating: Low to moderate.

Vaccine: Not yet routinely available in Ireland. Being tested in the US.

RUBELLA (German Measles)

Cause: A virus.

Infectivity: Highly contagious. Prior to immunisation parents used to organise 'rubella tea-parties', where little girls passed on the natural illness to one another.

Age-group: Any, but usually young children.

Features: A mild illness characterised by fever, fine red rash, swollen glands and occasionally pain in the joints.

Complications: Unusual in childhood. However, potentially very serious in pregnant women in the first six months of pregnancy. May result in foetal death, severe foetal damage, and deafness.

Severity rating: Low in small children, high in pregnant women.

Vaccine: A live, weakened virus. Very effective in preventing congenital (from birth) rubella syndrome.

HiB INVASIVE DISEASE

Cause: Haemophilus influenzae B, a common bacterium.

Infectivity: Fairly infectious. Spread by close contact.

Age-group: Infants and toddlers usually.

Features/
complications: Causes many different illnesses, including meningitis (inflammation of the brain lining), septicaemia (infection in the bloodstream), pneumonia, osteomyelitis (infection of bone), septic arthritis (infection of joint), epiglottitis (a serious form of croup), tracheitis (infection of the windpipe).

Severity rating: High.

Vaccine: Introduced in 1992. Very successful so far in reducing these serious diseases.

TETANUS

Cause: A bacterium in soil and manure entering wounds or puncture sites.

Age-group: All ages.

Features: 'Lock-jaw', severe muscle spasms, death.

Severity rating: High.

Vaccine: 95 per cent effective. Tetanus has been virtually eradicated in Irish children.

Infection	Incubation period (days)	Exclusion from school (days)
Measles	7-14	Four days from appearance of rash.
Rubella (German measles)	14-21	Four days from appearance of rash.
Varicella (chicken-pox)	10-24	Until rash becomes crusted.
Mumps	12-31	Seven days after swelling subsides.

Despite the widespread availability of vaccines, Ireland still has a fairly low rate of immunisation. The World Health Organisation recommends 90 to 95 per cent population immunisation. Ireland's immunisation rate is stuck at about 70 to 80 per cent. Immunisation uptakes of less than 70 per cent mean that diseases can still spread. Uptakes of 80 per cent mean that diseases are reasonably controlled and contained. Uptakes in excess of 90 to 95 per cent result in effective elimination of disease.

Denis G Gill MB, DCH, FRCPI is Professor of Paediatrics at the Royal College of Surgeons in Ireland, Dean of the Faculty of Paediatrics at the Royal College of Physicians of Ireland, and Paediatrician and Paediatric Nephrologist at the Children's Hospital, Temple Street, and Beaumont Hospital, Dublin.

SCHOOL DIFFICULTIES

PAUL ANDREWS SJ

A child who is unhappy at school can upset the whole family. Getting out of the house is a torture every morning, and doing the homework can be a major hassle every evening.

Psychologist and former headmaster Fr Paul Andrews describes some of the problems that children can have at school, and explains how understanding parents can do much to help them get through a difficult time.

REFUSING TO GO TO SCHOOL

Before 'school phobia' was identified as a condition, all persistent absence from school was labelled 'truancy'. With school phobia, the child is away from school for long periods, but the parents know where he is — usually at home. The reasons for his absence are a puzzle both to his parents and to his school. The child may say he is afraid of the teacher or afraid to go to school. At home he is happy, but when dragged to school he is miserable, fearful and likely to run home at the first opportunity, no matter what the consequences. What appears at first to be an understandable reluctance to face the tasks of school may turn into something quite formidable. The warning signs usually fall into the following categories:

School sickness: When a child says he is ill, his parents will generally be able, with the help of a thermometer, to discern how serious it is. The child may be suffering from 'school sickness'. Watch for signs of health, like eating a hearty breakfast or running to the door for the postman. Have a clear-cut regime for sickness: all day in bed, very quiet, no proper meals, no television, no friends to visit or phone. Suggest calling the doctor. If he is sick, the regime will help him to recover. Above all, ensure that being ill at home is generally dull and unrewarding.

Occasional refusing: Every now and then school becomes just too much for your child and you give him a day off, judging his fatigue or lassitude from your knowledge of his moods. If this happens regularly on a particular day, you may find that he is avoiding some weekly feature that daunts him, such as changing for PE.

Panicky refusing: This happens because the child has experienced some upset or failure that threw him completely, and he is afraid it will happen again: an accident in the toilets; perhaps doing something stupid in front of the class; an angry word from a teacher he had idolised, and so forth. When you give him a sympathetic ear, the story emerges, and it is usually possible to work round the problem with the teacher's help.

Firm and persistent refusing: The child resists going to school with all the strength he can muster, and with such vehemence that it seems a matter of life and death. His reasons (dislike of teacher, being annoyed by other children, feeling he cannot cope...) may have some basis, but they do not explain his terror. This is the more serious type of school phobia and may require the help of a child psychologist. First, however, listen to his fears and work through possible remedies. If he makes a scene leaving you at the school gate, have somebody else bring him to school. If he feels isolated, or overwhelmed by numbers, ask the teacher to find him a special friend for playtime. Do not ignore the problem or allow him to stay at home without a reason, or send in a spurious excuse to school. Above all, do not make unreal threats about sending him away or calling the gardaí. Unless there are very good reasons, do not change school. In most cases the problems will recur as strongly in the new school, and the child will have the additional problem of the loss of familiar friends and setting.

In helping a child with school phobia, it is best to get him back to school as soon as possible. The longer he stays out, the stronger will be the anxiety associated with school. It will require great strength of will in one or other parent to carry through the return to school, starting with gentle pressure and increasing it gradually. Two parallel approaches may well be needed: a parent working on the return to school, and a therapist listening to the child and sorting out the anxieties that triggered the school refusal.

Often, though not always, the issue is one of separation from the mother, and the trigger is a traumatic event that threatened someone close to the child. If this is the cause, then tackling a severe case of school refusal will involve pain for both child and parent.

THE CHILD WHO HAS NO FRIENDS

For the child who doesn't have friends, break times and lunch times can be sheer misery. A young child starting school can be helped by his mother or father befriending other parents at the school gate, and arranging for their children to get together outside school.

Older children often find themselves shut out by groups or gangs in the playground. While you cannot organise your child's social life — and to do so would slow down his social learning — you can tackle his misery on two fronts. First, by alerting the teacher, who can usually harness some good will in the other children to save your child from isolation. Secondly, by watching his behaviour with other children and listening to what his brothers and sisters say about him. For example, is he making himself unpopular? Perhaps he is so anxious to please that he invites snubs. Perhaps he is bossy and has to have his own way all the time. Perhaps he covers up his insecurity by clinging hard to teacher or by 'big talk' and boasting. A parent who observes and listens well can impart lessons in public relations at an early age that will never be forgotten.

BULLYING

School management boards now have guidelines to prevent and deal with cases of bullying. All teachers are aware of the danger, and can be called on to help tackle it. But every school still has its bullies: the friendless boy who finds that frightening another child is less lonely than having contact with nobody; the girl who has been put down at home and takes out her unhappiness on the weaker children at school.

There are natural victims too: friendless children who unconsciously encourage bullying as preferable to having no attention at all (they can be helped to make friends, as explained above); mamma's boys, dependent and over-protected, who have been able to manipulate their mother into fighting their battles for them; children who through no fault of their own are out of step with the rest, because they joined the class late, wear unusual clothes, or speak with an unusual accent; or children whose poor personal hygiene draws adverse attention — this can be quickly rectified by parents.

It is difficult for a child to tell you that he is being bullied; it makes him feel guilty and inadequate. So listen warmly, showing neither anger nor disappointment, but conveying a sense that the problem can be overcome. He must learn to walk tall, be confident enough to say 'No', hold his place in a queue when pushed out, demand his place on the swings, or his rights in the playground. He must also be ready to go on talking to you and his teacher if the bullying continues. Involve the teacher, school principal or playground supervisor, depending on who is able to offer practical help.

There are times when a child should put safety first and surrender money or whatever else is demanded, for example, when confronted by a vicious gang on the way home from school. When such an occurrence takes place he should be praised by his parents for his commonsense in that situation. Don't encourage a bullied child to fight back, beyond the requirements of self-defence. It can lead him into a cycle of violence beyond his powers to manage.

What about tackling the bully or his parents? This sort of thing can work, but only with adults who can resist getting into a fight with the other parents and are able to keep the encounter calm and discreet. The aim is to indicate clearly to the bully that you all know what is going on and are determined to put a stop to it.

THE CHILD WHO IS NOT WORKING

Why do children work at school? Younger children work because it pleases their parents and teachers. Older children (15+) work because they see the relevance of academic success to their future chances in life. In between, i.e. the first two or three years of secondary school, is a No Man's Land in terms of motivation.

The best way to motivate children is to give them some experience of success. If they start to do well in some area, like sport or music, they will learn how effort leads to reward, and there will usually be a spin-off in their schoolwork. Children learn little from failure, and their noses are sometimes rubbed in it by parents who are more in touch with their own anxieties than their children's needs. Contrive some way in which your child will feel himself moving forwards rather than backwards.

Through all the years of school, children respond consciously or unconsciously to their parents' expectations, and it helps if parents are aware of what they are doing. If they want more for their child than they achieved themselves, he may rebel; he wants to please, but he also wants to be himself, possibly in areas quite different from his parents' dreams. If at some level they expect him to fail, he probably will fail. If they see him as a prize bloom, for whom only the top awards are good enough, he may be so afraid of failing that he will not try at all.

Motivation to achieve grows where parents are warmly and intensely interested in all that the child does, but in a non-intrusive way. Anything he can do for himself, they let him do, and they show an encouraging but not uncritical interest in the results. They would rather see him try something alone and make mistakes from which he can learn, than do it perfectly with their help. Homework is his job, a way of learning how to work independently, and from the beginning his parents will stand back from the tackling of homework, though keeping a keen eye on the results.

You should consider the possibility that perhaps your child is not working or doing well at school because of some physical problem. Does he show signs of illness, of not getting enough sleep or food, or the wrong sort of food, or an undiagnosed condition of the glands, eyes, ears or digestive system? Usually the mother is the first to notice such conditions.

The reason could be simply that he is unable to cope with the work of the class. He may be genuinely too slow for a normal class, or have missed the foundations in one or more subjects, or have a specific difficulty with reading or spelling (see 'Dyslexia' below). If he is genuinely unable to cope with the work, he will probably react to it either by depressed withdrawal into himself, or by acting up in class and disturbing everyone.

Quite often the reason for idleness at school is an upset at home. Perhaps the child has overheard a shouting match between his parents, or resents a new baby, or feels in the shadow of a bright older sister or brother. His mind is in too much emotional turmoil to focus on classwork. Perceptive parents can usually pick out what the trouble is, and either talk it through, or support their child through a bad time, while letting the teacher know that he is under some stress.

Sometimes teachers comment that a child seems to have poor concentration. Usually this is only partly true. The child's mind may wander when faced with a page of sums or Irish grammar, but he can scan the TV programmes like lightning or spend hours playing video games with no sign of distraction. If he can do that, he has excellent powers of concentration, provided he is interested. There are, however, unfortunate hyperactive children who cannot keep their mind on one thing for more than thirty seconds, no matter how much they like it. (See chapter on 'Hyperactivity'.)

CHILDREN IN TROUBLE AT SCHOOL

If your child has run into trouble at primary school, there is a universally applied code of discipline that the school must observe in dealing with him. Suspension is a major sanction that is reserved for continuously disruptive pupils, or for a serious breach of discipline. The Board of Management may authorise the Principal to suspend a child from school for up to three days. If the trouble should develop to the point where expulsion is being considered, the school may not expel a child unless alternative arrangements are made for his enrolment at another suitable school in the locality.

At secondary level, there is such a variety of schools, most of them under private management, that it is not possible to indicate any generally binding pattern of discipline.

DYSLEXIA

There are many reasons why a child may have reading and writing difficulties, and these must be ruled out before a diagnosis of dyslexia can be made. The dyslexic child can be identified by the following factors:

- *Intelligence is average or above average.* If the child is slow in every area of learning, then it would be incorrect to treat him as having a specific reading difficulty.

- *His hearing and vision are normal.* If either of these are weak, then refer the physical defect to your doctor. Clearly a child who has impaired hearing or sight is going to find reading difficult.

- *There is no evidence of damage to the brain or nervous system,* eg cerebral palsy.

- *He has had the normal opportunities for schooling up to now.* A badly disrupted schooling in the first three years can account for poor reading, without the depressing assumption of dyslexia.

- *He had no marked emotional upset that pre-dated his reading difficulty.* Was he an upset child before he ever looked at a book? Perhaps that upset interfered with his early learning and accounts for his problem with reading.

Dyslexics are children with normal intelligence, hearing and eyesight, with no brain damage, who seem emotionally stable and have received an appropriate education, but cannot read even the simplest new word, nor use individual letters as the building blocks of words, whether in reading or in spelling. They are often confused about right and left, and consequently about telling the time, tying bows, and placing digits in arithmetic.

The term 'dyslexia' denotes a condition that can be helped but not cured. Early recognition is important. The term is often used loosely, sometimes by parents of children who are simply slow in reading, spelling and everything else. The dyslexic child, however, is quick at picking up information that is not in written form. The fact that reading and writing dominate nearly everything he does in school is a constant source of frustration for him.

Researchers are uncovering more about dyslexia all the time. It is more common among boys than girls and it usually comes to notice at fifth class level, when normal readers become fluent and hungry for books. It would seem to run in families (Chromosome 15 is suspected of carrying the weakness, which is transmitted more easily by mothers than fathers). Much of this is speculative, however, and not very useful to your child.

It is important not to label your child as dyslexic too quickly, as there are many milder reading problems that can be overcome with skilled tuition. If he is found to be truly dyslexic, then some long-term strategies are needed.

Because of his reading and writing difficulties, he may need help in learning things off by heart.

His handwriting will almost certainly be chaotic, and will remain a labour for him. If you or the school can afford it, teach him to master the keyboard of a word-processor, and to use the built-in spelling check, so that when something needs to be presented well, he can print it. He may develop a strength in computers, because children whose language skills are below average can still be highly competent in learning the operational sequences needed for computers. For other learning, educational TV can be of help.

You will know better than anyone how to avoid situations where the child's problem can make him look stupid. When eating out, read the menu to him without comment. Avoid leaving written messages for him; many families will have a tape recorder, and he should learn to use this for passing on messages, planning stories and essays, and possibly even doing exams in school.

Basic learning cannot be a pleasure for the dyslexic child; you can anticipate unusual levels of frustration, and will have to work to support his motivation all the way through school. Build up the areas (possibly music or computers) where he can show his gifts.

Severe dyslexia remains a problem even after school, so your child may have to be steered towards training and work that uses his strengths and does not require a lot of reading. Those who mark public examinations may make allowance for dyslexia, and this should be planned in good time through the school. Even if your dyslexic child gets a good Leaving Certificate, as a result of sheer hard work, he should not be pushed into a job where he will still depend to any great extent on writing and reading.

EXAMINATION PHOBIA

In Ireland as in other European countries, about 15 per cent of the school population are just no good when it comes to public examinations, and it is wise to spare them the ordeal. For the others, formal examinations are the passport to almost every career; they are unavoidable. The Leaving Certificate in particular carries a heavy burden of decision for every candidate. The burden is placed there by society, not by the school, which can do little to change the system, though it can help students to beat it.

Some students are frightened or depressed by exams, even to the point of suicide, often seeing more in the exam than just a set of questions. For them it feels like the Day of Judgement, or Big Brother peering into their mind and tut-tutting over the sorry mess inside. When the exam course is viewed as a whole, the child is terrified, but when he focuses on a limited section of a subject, he masters it competently. Panic arises only at the thought of being examined on the entirety of the course.

Parents and teachers can help by keeping the child's attention focused on the parts rather than the whole, and by repeated rehearsal of the details of the exam so that he is familiar with the colour and lay-out of each paper, the type of questions commonly asked, and the range of choice. As the exam draws near he can be further helped by a stable routine at home, which refuses to be sucked into his nervousness, and by a concern for his physical well-being, his sleep, appetite and exercise. Panicky people infect those around them. At this final hurdle, as in all the preceding crises of his childhood, he will learn more from the calmness of his parents than from their arguments.

Useful address

Association for Children and Adults with Learning Disabilities, 1 Suffolk Street, Dublin 2. Tel. (01) 6790276.

Paul Andrews is a Jesuit priest and psychologist. Since 1977 he has been Director of Saint Declan's School and Child Guidance Centre, Northumberland Road, Dublin 4.

SKIN CONDITIONS

DR ROSEMARIE WATSON

Our skin fulfils all kinds of useful functions. It protects us from infections and damage by sunlight, and it holds in water and chemicals. It also helps to regulate the body's temperature, and it helps us feel pain, touch, temperature and itch. Because skin conditions are visible, they can be diagnosed very quickly, but this visibility also means that skin conditions can cause great psychological as well as physical hurt.

Dr Rosemarie Watson, a consultant dermatologist, describes the most common skin problems, from birthmarks to eczema, and athlete's foot to head lice.

BIRTHMARKS

Birthmarks can be divided into two main types, vascular birthmarks and moles (congenital naevi).

Vascular birthmarks (strawberry marks, etc)

Vascular birthmarks, caused by an excess of small blood vessels in a localised area of skin, are the most common, occurring in 10 per cent of all infants under one year of age. The strawberry birthmark (haemangioma) typically appears within the first four weeks of life, and enlarges over weeks or months to reach a stable size, after which it goes into a phase of healing and begins to fade. These skin lesions are more common in girls and in very premature infants. Fifty per cent will have faded by age five and 70 per cent by age seven. They are called strawberry marks because of their bright red colour. Some, however, are found more deeply in the skin, have a bluish tinge and take longer to clear. They can occur on any body site and generally require no treatment, unless they are interfering with feeding, obstructing the airway or interfering with vision. Treatment in these extremely unusual situations is usually in the form of cortisone. These haemangiomas may occasionally bleed, in which case firm pressure should be applied over the area for five to ten minutes, and repeated if necessary. If the bleeding does not stop with pressure, you should consult your family doctor or the casualty department of your local hospital. The vast majority heal with minimal scarring, although there may be some slight thinning of the skin in the area.

Salmon patches are also common, appearing as a flat, dull, pink area on the nape of the neck or on the forehead, between the eyes. No treatment is necessary, as more than 90 per cent of those on the face fade by one year of age. A small percentage of those on the nape of the neck persist, but are eventually hidden by hair.

Port-wine stains are the least common form of vascular lesion, affecting 0.3 per cent of infants. They may appear on any part of the body, but the face and neck are the most common sites. They are usually flat and pink in infancy, but tend to darken to a dull red or purple hue, and may become thickened. Until recently the only solution was to try to camouflage them with cosmetics. However, the pulse dye laser has been a major advance in treatment: a laser beam destroys the vessels in the port-wine stain with almost no scarring. It may take numerous treatments over many months, but cosmetic results are excellent. Children may be treated as early as infancy onwards.

Moles

Moles can be divided into congenital (present at birth) or acquired. One per cent of all infants have congenital moles, which fall into three groups according to their size. Small congenital moles are those less than 1.5cm ($\frac{1}{2}$in) in diameter, medium-size congenital moles are those greater than 1.5cm ($\frac{1}{2}$in) but less than 10cm (4in), while giant or large congenital moles are those measuring in excess of 10cm (4in).

Small congenital moles appear as light tan to brown areas on the skin. They tend not to change over time, except for the occasional appearance of coarse dark hair. Larger congenital moles may have an uneven, rough surface.

Acquired moles, on the other hand, usually appear from age two to three years onwards, and are generally less than 1cm in diameter. They may continue to grow as the child grows, and may become elevated in the centre. Research would suggest that there is a small increased risk of melanoma, a form of skin cancer, in people with congenital moles. This risk would appear to be somewhat higher in the large to giant congenital moles.

With any mole, you should bring your child to a doctor if you notice a change in growth pattern or colour, particularly if this is restricted to only one area of the mole, or if there is a history of bleeding or prolonged itching. In such cases it may be advisable to have the mole removed by surgery.

ECZEMA (ATOPIC DERMATITIS)

Eczema affects between 5 and 10 per cent of children. It is an inflammation of the skin, and it can cause an intense itch. It is thought to be hereditary and is often associated with asthma or hayfever. Sixty per cent of eczema begins in the first year of life, and 85 per cent of children with eczema develop the condition before the age of five. In very young children the usual locations are the face and neck, arms and legs, tops of the hands, and feet. After the age of three the eczema tends to be located in the folds of the elbow and behind the knees.

Itch can be triggered by sudden changes in temperature or by irritants such as wool, soap and detergents. The skin becomes dry, red and coarse, and on occasions may develop cracks (fissures) and open sores. Weeping and crusting of the skin is usually a sign of infection, a common complication in eczema. Constant scratching causes damage to the barrier function of the skin, and the loss of water and resulting dryness aggravates the itch. Eczema tends to flare when babies are teething and it often flares in the winter months when the air is dry and humidity is low. Some children find summertime more troublesome, when sweating may aggravate the itch.

Treatment

There is no single treatment for eczema. Several areas need attention. The most important aspect of the treatment is hydration of the skin. Daily baths are recommended to keep the skin clean and free from crusts and scales. Bathing also adds much-needed moisture to the skin. A bath oil emollient (skin softener) should be added to the bath water and the child should soak in the water for at least ten minutes. The majority of soaps dry the skin and should be avoided. Ask your pharmacist for suitable soap substitutes.

After the bath, pat the skin gently until it is almost dry, and apply an emollient cream to moisturise the skin. Ideally emollients should be applied three times daily. If the skin is very dry, the child should also be bathed three times daily.

Steroid preparations are most useful in controlling the inflammation. If a steroid cream or ointment has been recommended by your doctor, it should be applied sparingly to the red itchy areas. Many parents worry about the side-effects of steroid creams. Generally, side-effects such as thinning of the skin are caused by the misuse of strong steroid creams, which are not usually prescribed for children. The long-term use of a mild steroid cream, such as one per cent hydrocortisone, applied sparingly to small areas once or twice daily, is safe.

Emollients are the usual form of treatment for facial eczema, but if they don't work, one per cent hydrocortisone can be used, preferably for brief periods.

If these methods do not control the itching, an antihistamine medicine may give further relief. This medication may be given three or four times daily, and is most useful at bedtime when the heat of the bed sometimes triggers a child's itching. It is also a good idea to keep the bedroom cool. If your child's eczema is not responding to the usual treatments, there may be infection present, and antibiotics may be needed.

Tar is another valuable topical treatment in eczema. This can be applied in the form of an ointment or as a tar-medicated bandage.

Other treatments sometimes used are Evening Primrose Oil and, in more severe eczema, ultraviolet-light therapy.

Recent research also suggests that some powerful drugs (such as cyclosporin) that affect the immune system may improve eczema. These are not without significant side-effects and should be reserved for children with severe eczema.

New in the list of treatments is a Chinese herbal diet, but this needs further assessment to evaluate its long-term safety.

Allergies and eczema

Children with eczema have hypersensitive skin, so they may react to many environmental allergens (allergy-causing substances) such as grass pollen, cat and dog fur, house-dust mites and feathers. It is wise to avoid these substances.

Most parents are anxious to know if their child's eczema is caused by a food allergy. In over 90 per cent of children food allergies play no role in their eczema. However, a small percentage may react to certain foods, in particular eggs, cow's milk, fish and peanuts. The allergy is usually diagnosed by the parent noticing swelling of the lips, hives, or a significant flare of the eczema, usually within two to three hours of taking the offending food. Allergy tests, including skin and blood tests, are generally not helpful, as they produce many false positive reactions.

The good news is that the vast majority of children grow out of eczema. If a child has severe eczema, she may be prone to dermatitis of the hands later in life. For these reasons, it is wise to counsel children in the teenage years against becoming interested in occupations that involve a lot of wet work, for example, hairdressing, nursing, etc.

SEBORRHOEIC DERMATITIS

Infantile seborrhoeic dermatitis is a common skin condition of unknown cause, characterised by scaling and redness of the skin, particularly affecting the eyebrows, ears, scalp (cradle cap) and body folds, notably the under arms and nappy area. The rash is not particularly itchy, and most cases clear within three to four weeks, even without specific treatment. Some cases can last up to six months. This condition is managed in a similar way to eczema, with frequent baths, emollients, and steroid cream for red, inflamed areas. Cradle cap can be cleared by rubbing olive oil into the scalp and washing with a mild tar shampoo.

PSORIASIS

Psoriasis is a common condition in both adults and children, and tends to run in families. It is the cause of approximately 4 per cent of skin conditions in those under the age of sixteen. There are several different kinds of psoriasis, but the usual types in children are plaque psoriasis and guttate psoriasis.

Plaque psoriasis results in red scaly patches, typically located on the elbows, knees, scalp, belly button and buttocks, and in the nappy area in young children. The nails may also be involved, with thickening and surface pits.

In guttate psoriasis, small red scaly patches appear all over the body, often rather abruptly. This form of psoriasis is sometimes seen a few weeks after a streptococcal infection. Occasionally, treatment of a previously undiagnosed streptococcal infection can lead to improvement in the psoriasis.

Most cases of psoriasis are treated with tar preparations or steroid creams. Anthralin (dithranol) and Calcipotriol, which are used more frequently with adults, may be prescribed in severe cases. Sunlight is very beneficial, and most children improve during the summer months. Occasionally, ultraviolet light may be given as a treatment in hospital. Because ultraviolet light over long periods is damaging to the skin, sunbeds are not advised. Hospitalisation may be considered in severe cases, when intensive tar treatments are required. Injury to the skin can bring out psoriasis, therefore it is advisable to avoid tight constrictive clothing and repeated injury to the skin. However, a child's activities should not be restricted to the point where this interferes with her psychological or social development, so children should be encouraged to attend regular classes and engage in most activities. Adolescents especially may find it difficult to accept psoriasis, since they see it as disfiguring and unattractive. They should be encouraged to verbalise their feelings so they can learn to cope better with their chronic skin condition. Psoriasis tends to wax and wane, and treatment can lead to long remissions. Thankfully, it is not contagious, and most cases of psoriasis in childhood are well controlled with creams and ointments.

INFECTIONS

Impetigo

Impetigo is a very common skin condition caused by a bacterial infection. Yellow, weeping, crusted areas appear on the skin, at times amounting to blisters. Impetigo is contagious but is easily treated with either an antibiotic cream or an oral antibiotic.

Ringworm

Ringworm infections are caused by a fungus, usually acquired by contact with other humans or animals. When the scalp is affected, it may cause hair loss. Ringworm is easily identified by the ring-shaped patches it causes. When limited to small areas these can be treated by an antifungal cream, but infection of the scalp and more widespread areas requires treatment with an oral antifungal drug such as Griseofulvin.

Athlete's foot

Athlete's foot is seen more often now that sneakers are in fashion. It flourishes in a hot, humid environment, and causes scaling and itching between the toes and on the foot. It is treatable with an antifungal cream. Even if there is no fungal infection, wearing sneakers continually can cause scaling and fissuring or cracks on the soles of the feet. The skin can become shiny in appearance. It is important to keep the child out of sneakers as much as possible and to use moisturisers frequently. Occasionally, a one per cent hydrocortisone cream or tar preparations are required to keep it under control. Eczema and psoriasis can also affect children's feet.

Cold Sores (Herpes Simplex)

Over 90 per cent of the population have been exposed to the *herpes simplex* virus by the time they reach their teens. Attacks can occur at any age and are spread by skin contact. The first attack is often the worst, and may be associated with fever and enlarged lymph glands in the neck. It is most often seen on the lips, but may occur at other sites on the face or body. The skin is red, and in the early phases has small fluid-filled blisters, which burst and form a crust. This condition tends to recur and is aggravated by infections (eg colds, pneumonia), sunlight, wind and stress. Acyclovir cream

(Zovirax) can help speed up the healing in those prone to recurrent attacks. It must be applied as soon as the symptoms begin.

Warts

Not many children escape through childhood without getting warts. They are caused by a papilloma virus infection of the skin and are perfectly harmless. They may infect any area of the skin, and 70 per cent will disappear without treatment within two years.

The presence of warts in the genital area in young children sometimes raises the possibility of childhood sexual abuse, but research has shown that this is rarely the cause. The more frequent methods of spreading genital warts are by transmission from the mother's birth canal, often resulting in warts in the child before age two, and from hand warts on the child herself, or on her minders, transmitted during nappy changes and so forth.

In general, no treatment is necessary for warts, but if they become troublesome they can be treated with salicylic acid preparations, available from your pharmacy (eg Duofilm, Salatac). Cryotherapy (liquid nitrogen), which freezes the warts, can be used by your doctor, but causes discomfort and is best avoided in younger children. Genital warts should be referred to your doctor for treatment.

Molluscum contagiosum

Molluscum is another common skin infection caused by the pox virus. It is characterised by pearly bumps on the skin, which often have a central core. There may be several present, ranging from pinhead size to several millimetres. No treatment is required as they heal spontaneously. If they become infected an antibiotic may be needed. Occasionally doctors will use Cryotherapy (liquid nitrogen) to treat molluscum, but nature is likely to be the best healer.

VIRAL RASHES

Viral rashes are extremely common in children and can be caused by over fifty different viruses. The majority of viral rashes take the form of red spots all over the skin, and get better over a week or two. (See chapter on 'Infectious Diseases'.)

INFESTATIONS

Scabies

Scabies is an intensely itchy rash caused by a tiny mite or bug that lives in the skin. It is almost impossible to see it without magnification. It usually affects the hands, wrists, between the fingers, and genital area. In young babies scabies typically affects the palms, soles and underarm area, and may affect the scalp. It tends to spare the face and scalp in older children.

Scabies is contagious, and is transmitted by close personal contact. All members of the family, including babysitters, should be treated at the same time. If the baby is in a creche, the owner of the creche should be informed. Scabies is not often spread by clothes or bedding, so there is no need to sterilise these; they can simply be machine-washed after treatment.

Treatment consists of applying mite-killing medication to the skin. Directions should be followed exactly. The medicine should be applied to the entire skin, from the neck down, not just to the itching areas. Young babies may need the scalp treated. Rub the medicine thoroughly into the child's hands and wrists, and do not wash the hands for eight hours. When the baby's nappy is changed, the medicine should be reapplied. It should not be applied for longer than directed, or more frequently than directed, as it will irritate the skin. It is also absorbed through the skin, and too much may be toxic.

Treatment usually results in improvement of the itch and rash over two to six weeks, but it is important for parents to be aware that the itching and the rash may continue even after all the mites have been killed. The rash is largely an allergy to the mites and is called post-scabetic dermatitis. Post-scabetic dermatitis is not scabies, and may be treated with frequent baths, moisturisers, antihistamines and a steroid cream if necessary.

Head lice

Head lice is a troublesome condition because it is easily spread, particularly within schools. You may first notice your child scratching her head, and closer scrutiny may reveal nits stuck to the hairs. These are the whitish to sandy coloured empty shells of eggs that have hatched; newly laid eggs are more difficult to see and may be tan to coffee coloured or darker. The head lice are about two to three millimetres in size when they are fully grown.

Some people feel that head lice are an indication of poor hygiene or parental neglect. Nothing could be further from the truth. They are caused simply by close contact with another individual who has head lice.

The treatment consists of a special shampoo, usually Lindane or Prioderm. The recommended treatment time is less than ten minutes. You can use a fine comb or your fingernails to remove nits. Children should be encouraged not to share combs, brushes, towels or other items that come in contact with the head. There is now a shampoo on the market that acts as a lice-repellent. It will not completely prevent reinfection, but may be a helpful addition if you feel your child is likely to be re-exposed.

ALOPECIA (HAIR LOSS)

There are four main causes of alopecia in childhood:

Telogen effluvium: This is a form of generalised hair loss that is likely to occur approximately two to three months after a severe illness, surgery or high fever. In this situation the hair falls out by the roots, and will usually grow back again in a few months.

Ringworm of the scalp: Ringworm can be associated with patchy areas of hair loss and dandruff-like scales on the surface of the scalp.

Alopecia areata: This is an uncommon condition that can affect both adults and children. The hair is usually lost in round patches. The surface of the scalp is smooth, without dryness or scales. One or several areas of the scalp may be involved. Very rarely, all scalp hair may be lost in this condition. Sometimes there is a family history of thyroid conditions. The cause of this type of hair loss is unknown, but in well over 90 per cent of cases the hair grows again without any treatment after several weeks or months. Steroid or Dithranol creams or cortisone injections can be used on occasion to encourage regrowth.

Hormone or vitamin deficiency: Deficiency of certain hormones or vitamins may occasionally cause hair loss. Your doctor may wish to check your child's blood for anaemia or an underactive thyroid gland. Hair loss due to these deficiencies should reverse with treatment.

HIVES (URTICARIA)

Hives are red, itchy weals which can occur on any area of the body. Sometimes they may be associated with swelling of the lips, and very occasionally swelling of the tongue or throat. Hives are common and may be caused by allergies to food, notably eggs, peanuts, dairy products, wheat and soya. However, the majority of hives are not caused by food allergies; they may be caused by viral infections, insect bites, grass or pet fur allergy, or by an infection such as sinusitis or dental abscess. No underlying cause is found in over 50 per cent of patients with hives. The treatment is antihistamine medication and cooling lotions, which may be applied to the skin.

If your child shows difficulty breathing or appears to be choking during an episode of hives, you should bring her to a doctor immediately. The majority of hives clear within four to six weeks, but in a few children they may persist for some months.

PROTECTING THE SKIN

We can all play a part in preventing the skin cancer melanoma in our children by giving them good advice regarding sun protection: cover up, wear a hat and use a sunblock sun-protection factor of fifteen or higher when outdoors. Research has shown that over 50 per cent of a lifetime's sun exposure is acquired before the age of twenty. Protecting our children will go a long way towards preventing skin cancers in the future.

Useful addresses

Psoriasis Association of Ireland *and* National Eczema Society, both based at Carmichael House, North Brunswick St, Dublin 7. Tel. (01) 8735702.

Dr Rosemarie Watson FRCPI, FACP is Consultant Dermatologist at Our Lady's Hospital for Sick Children, Crumlin, Dublin.

SLEEP PROBLEMS AND BEDWETTING

DR CAROL FITZPATRICK

It can take many months before a new baby settles down to something resembling a normal sleep pattern and his distracted parents manage to have an occasional uninterrupted night.

Consultant child psychiatrist Dr Carol Fitzpatrick advises parents on how to survive those early days, and how to cope with some of the other sleep problems, including bedwetting and night terrors, that can affect older children.

Sleep that knits up the ravell'd sleeve of care,
The death of each day's life, sore labour's bath,
Balm of hurt minds, great nature's second course,
Chief nourisher in life's feast.

Shakespeare's *Macbeth*

Shakespeare's description of sleep as the great restorer will ring true with parents of young children. Young babies wake at night to be fed, while older infants and toddlers frequently go through phases of night-waking and crying which can tax the stamina of the most patient parent. It is very rare for young children to suffer ill-effects from 'not getting enough sleep', as children of all ages vary widely in the amount of sleep they need, and young children who need more sleep than they are getting at night compensate during the day with naps and snoozes. However, the luxury of a daytime nap is usually impossible for busy mothers and fathers, and children's night-time sleeping problems are a common cause of fatigue, irritability and strained relationships in parents. It is easy to see how a vicious cycle can develop, with night-time sleep problems leading to difficult relations between children and parents, which may in turn lead to further sleep problems.

NORMAL SLEEP PATTERNS IN CHILDHOOD

There is tremendous individual variation both in the amount of sleep required by healthy children and in their sleep patterns. 'Easy' babies in our culture are those who from the early weeks of life fall into a pattern of regular, predictable periods of sleeping and wakefulness, and who sleep through the night from an early age. By the time they are three months old, about 70 per cent of babies are sleeping through the night, and by one year of age about 90 per cent are doing so. It would however be more correct to say that these babies are 'getting through the night without waking their parents', as studies of the electrical activity of the brain (electro-encephalographic or EEG studies) have shown that the vast majority of babies, infants and children wake at least once during the night.

What differentiates children with night-time waking problems from other children is the fact that they appear to be unable to settle back to sleep without the intervention of a parent.

Studies of the electrical activity of the brain during sleep show two different types of sleep, quiet sleep and rapid eye movement (REM) sleep, which alternate in cycles. During REM sleep there is a reduction in muscle tone, rapid changes in pulse rate, blood pressure and rate of breathing, as well as bursts of rapid eye movements. It is thought that most dreaming occurs during REM sleep, and young babies have proportionally much more REM sleep than older children and adults. A parent observing a baby in a state of REM sleep may mistakenly think that the muscle twitches and changes in the rate of breathing mean that the baby is restless and not having a proper sleep. This is not the case, as what they are seeing are the physical signs of a normal phase of sleep, in which the child is probably dreaming.

NIGHT-TIME CRYING

Problems in this area fall into two broad categories: difficulties in settling down to sleep, and night-time waking. If either of these problems occurs out of the blue in infants who have previously been good sleepers, the parent needs to look for a cause and, if possible, remedy it. For example, has the household routine been disrupted for any reason, or is the infant sickening for something? There is usually some explanation for a sudden onset of sleep problems.

There is, however, a large group of infants who habitually find it hard to settle at night, or who wake repeatedly during the night and cry until reassured by a parent, and who start crying again as soon as the parent leaves the room. For the infant who is difficult to settle it often helps to have a consistent pre-sleep routine. The time before going to sleep should be a period of progressively settling down, in which the routine of feeding, changing, maybe a cuddle or a story, is inevitably followed by the parent saying goodnight and withdrawing. It is unwise to get into the habit even with very young babies of keeping them downstairs until they are asleep, or allowing them to fall asleep in your arms, as this habit can be very hard to break once it has been established.

Sleeping medications for infants and young children are not to be recommended. Over-the-counter medications are widely used by parents of young children with sleep problems and may have a role to play in a very short-term crisis situation, but they will not solve well-established sleeping problems, and their long-term use is not advised.

Waking at night and difficulty in settling are best dealt with using a behavioural approach. The most effective behavioural approach is a 'systematic ignoring'. This requires careful planning, and agreement between both parents that it is worth trying and persisting with. After tucking up the child at bedtime, the parent leaves the room and resolves not to go back in until the child is asleep, come what may. When the child wakes at night, the parent ignores him. Obviously the parent must be sure at all times that the child is physically all right, but any 'checking' should be done quickly, and ideally without being seen. The first few nights will be traumatic for everyone, and it is worth warning the neighbours. Many parents worry that they will cause their child untold future emotional damage by using such an approach, but there is no evidence that this is the case. Indeed, it is probably much more damaging for the infant to have an ill-tempered, exhausted parent caring for him during the day, than it is to cry himself to sleep for a few nights. The value of this systematic ignoring is that if parents are able to stick to it, it is generally only necessary for three or four nights.

Not all parents can carry through with this strategy. Some feel it is too cruel, while others become so upset themselves that it leads to rows and fighting between parents, which may be worse than the original crying-baby problem. For such parents another approach that may prove successful is that called 'scheduled awakenings'. This is based on the fact that most babies who wake at night do so at a particular and fairly constant time or times. If the infant is woken briefly about thirty minutes before the time when he would wake naturally, he will often settle to sleep again after a few minutes and not wake at his usual waking time. In order to be successful these strategies must involve careful planning, discussion and the assent and support of both parents.

Many parents, when they are in a cycle of broken nights and fraught days with infants, feel that they cannot do anything differently and become very helpless. It is worth seeking the advice of your general practitioner or public health nurse if this is the case.

NIGHTMARES

These are frightening dreams that occur in the rapid eye movement (REM) phase of sleep. The child wakes up in an anxious state, but knows where he is and is able to relate the content of the dream that was upsetting him so much. Virtually all children experience at least occasional nightmares. They occur most frequently about the age of five to six years, although most people continue to experience nightmares occasionally throughout childhood and in adult life.

The child who is experiencing very frequent nightmares may be either over-stimulated or under stress. Over-stimulation may be due to watching exciting or terrifying television programmes or videos. Young children may be under stress for a variety of reasons, such as changes in routine, parental rows or parental ill-health. With older children it is important to consider sources of stress outside of the home, such as bullying at school.

NIGHT TERRORS

Night terrors are different from nightmares, and are much more frightening. In a night terror the child who has been sound asleep sits up abruptly in bed, screams and appears to be terrified. He seems to be awake with his eyes open, but it is impossible to make contact with him or to reassure him. The child often appears to be 'seeing things', typically frightening monsters or people with knives. Sometimes the child jumps out of bed and runs around the house in a state of tremendous anxiety. During this phase the child is inconsolable and often does not seem to know where he is or recognise those closest to him.

Night terrors may be more terrifying for parents as they can recall the episode the following morning, whereas the child usually does not. Many parents fear that their child is 'going mad', or that the night terrors are a sign of deep disturbance. They can be reassured that neither of these fears is true. We do not know what causes night terrors, nor why some children are more susceptible to them than others, but we do know that if the child appears otherwise untroubled during the day, they are not a sign of deep disturbance. Children with a tendency to night terrors often seem to get them when they are physically unwell, or going through a period of minor change or stress (eg changing schools). Most children grow out of night terrors, and they are rare in adult life.

Children with infrequent night terrors do not need any special treatment. The best way to manage the night terror is to be with the child to make sure he does not harm himself, but do not try to wake the child. In any case, it is usually impossible to do so, and if you shake him this may be incorporated into the night terror and interpreted by him as further evidence that he is being attacked. It is best not to quiz the child next morning about his night terror, as the anxiety that parents feel may be quickly transmitted to the child and may make night terrors more likely. A casual enquiry as to how he slept or if he had a bad dream gives him the opportunity to talk about his night terror, should he remember fragments of it, as he sometimes will.

Most night terrors occur within the first hour and a half of going to sleep, as they occur in a particular phase of sleep, and children who are having regular and frequent night terrors usually do so at a fixed length of time from when they go to sleep. This fact has led to the development of a simple but effective treatment strategy which involves charting the night terrors for the first few nights, noting what time the child goes to sleep and at what time the night terror occurs. Once the pattern is established, the parent wakes the child fifteen minutes before the anticipated night terror. The child usually goes back to sleep rapidly and does not suffer a night terror on that night. This treatment works because it disrupts the stage of sleep during which the child has the night terror. It is worth trying with children who are having repeated and regular night terrors. It should be combined with some thought and consideration as to what, if any, daytime stress might be contributing to the child's night terrors.

Another useful approach to the treatment of frequent and regular night terrors is the use of a small dose of an anti-depressant such as Imipramine for two to three weeks. We do not know how this acts in reducing night terrors, but it is not due to the anti-depressant action of the medication, as the dose used is very much smaller than that which is used in the treatment of depressive disorders. It probably acts by altering in some way the pattern of sleep.

BEDWETTING

Bedwetting is a common problem. Most children become dry at night somewhere between the ages of two and three, but about a third of normal children are still wetting the bed at night by the age of three, and by the age of five years about one tenth of children wet by night. By eight years of age about one child in twenty-five wets the bed regularly, and this falls to about one in a hundred by the age of fourteen years. Boys are more likely to wet the bed than girls.

The amount of distress this problem causes to the child and parent varies a great deal from family to family. In families where there is a history of bedwetting in other children, or where the parents wet the bed themselves as children, bedwetting is often viewed as something that the child will grow out of, almost a normal part of childhood, and not something that causes great distress. In other families bedwetting is a source of enormous tension, leading to embarrassment and shame on the child's part, and is often a cause of conflict between child and parents.

Bedwetting is usually due to slow maturation of the nervous system functions that control the bladder. Sometimes stresses in the child's environment that occur around the time the child would normally be developing bladder control seem to interfere with the child acquiring bladder control and can lead to persistence of bedwetting. Some children who have achieved bladder control at the usual age of two or three years lose that control following an upset or change in their routine. The birth of a younger brother or sister can often cause an upset for a toddler, and can lead to bedwetting, and to additional strain on parents coping with a new baby. This type of bedwetting is often shortlived and responds best to plenty of tender loving care during the day, while ignoring the bedwetting itself.

Occasionally bedwetting has an identifiable physical cause, such as a urinary tract infection, so it is advisable to have your child checked by your family doctor, who will carry out an examination of the urine to detect infection and will advise if other tests are necessary.

Management of bedwetting

It is always advisable to consider if the child has any stresses, such as frequent parental rows, school difficulties, teasing within the family or at school. (See chapter on 'School Difficulties'.) If the parent feels that there are problems that may have contributed to the bedwetting, it is worth trying to sort these out. However, in many cases there are no identifiable causes. One practical commonsense measure in dealing with bedwetting is to put a plastic cover over the mattress. A child aged from three to five may be helped by making as little fuss as possible around wet nights, combined with liberal praise for dry nights. Punishment does not work and is liable to make the problem worse. With an older child, of five to nine years, it is a good idea to make a calendar, with a space for each night into which the child places a star for each dry night. This is combined with a reward for perhaps two or three dry nights in a row. When rewarding the child, it is important not to use time periods that are likely to fail, such as in September promising them a large Christmas present if dry beds are maintained between then and Christmas.

Lifting the child and bringing him to the toilet before the parent retires to bed helps some children. While there is no scientific evidence to show that restricting a child's intake of fluids in the evening is effective, many parents like to try this, and it may make the child feel that he is contributing to an improvement in his problem if it actually works.

For older children a night-trainer alarm may prove very useful. It consists of a small pad placed in the child's pyjamas which, when it becomes wet, sets off a buzzer alarm and wakes the child. The child must then dry the pad, change the wet pyjamas and wet sheets and reset the alarm system before going back to sleep. In practice very few children have the motivation to do this on their own and do need their parents' help. It is actually quite a lot of hard work, but is useful with many older children. The night-trainer works by establishing a reflex whereby the child over a few weeks comes to wake up earlier and earlier during the actual wetting, and eventually before he wets. Night-trainers cost about seventy pounds and are available from hospital equipment supply shops. Many general practices and paediatric departments in hospitals will rent them out for a small fee.

There are now a variety of medications to help with bedwetting. Most of them suppress the wetting while the child is taking the medication, but the problem frequently recurs when the medication is stopped. They are very useful for special occasions, such as when a child is going on a school trip or on holidays. Medication can be used in combination with star charts, and sometimes the child gets a great boost in confidence by achieving dryness, which may last after the medication is discontinued. The use of medication is best discussed with your family doctor.

Some children are very embarrassed by their bedwetting, and it is a source of major anxiety to them, while others seem unaffected by it. How bedwetting is dealt with depends on your own and your child's reaction to it. But be consoled — the vast majority of children grow out of it with time.

WHERE TO GO FOR HELP

As most sleep difficulties are so common, it is often worth talking the problem over with friends who may have been through the same situation themselves and may be able to advise you. Problems with the under threes can be discussed with your public health nurse. You should not think that any problem is too trivial to discuss with your family doctor. Occasionally your GP may suggest referral to a paediatrician, a child psychologist or a child psychiatrist. Many parents do not seek help because they feel the problem is a trivial one and they should be able to deal with it on their own. However, if your child's night-time difficulty is causing stress that spills over into the day and is starting to affect your relationship with your child, it is definitely worth seeking help.

Dr Carol Fitzpatrick MD, FRCPI, MRC, Psych is Consultant Child Psychiatrist at Our Lady's Hospital for Sick Children, Crumlin, Dublin. She is also Consultant to the St John of God Child and Family Centres, Dublin.

SPEECH AND LANGUAGE

DR MARIE DE MONTFORT

The vast majority of children learn to talk with apparently little effort, so long as they have normal intelligence and hearing, and are in a stimulating environment in which language can flourish.

Dr Marie de Montfort is Director of the School of Clinical Speech and Language Studies, Trinity College, Dublin, the only centre in the country for training speech and language therapists. She explains how parents can help their children to develop good communication skills, and how they can recognise the common speech and language disorders.

STAGES OF NORMAL DEVELOPMENT

Most children develop their communication skills according to a set pattern, but the speed at which they develop can vary, even within the same family. There are usually parallels between the stages at which a child learns to walk, and the stages of language development.

- When a child is able to pull himself up to standing position, he is at the 'babbling' stage of speech development.

- When the child can crawl easily and stand alone, he can say a few words — this usually happens when he is about a year old.

- When the child starts to walk — at around eighteen months — he can use about twenty words and can understand approximately eighty.

- When the child can climb the stairs, he can use phrases — at about two-and-a-half years.

However, 'communication' commences long before the child learns to speak. For example, when you play with a baby and make cooing sounds, the child in turn responds with his own sounds. This becomes a game and continues for some time, just like a conversation. From approximately six months the child begins to derive meaning from your intonation.

Research has shown that the initial sounds a child makes are not influenced by what he hears around him. A baby will make the same babbling sounds whether he belongs to an English-speaking or a Japanese-speaking family. By nine to ten months the child begins to imitate specifically the sounds made to him by adults.

Children (and adults) will always understand more words than they use. The first meaningful word is usually said at around twelve months. Following this, vocabulary appears to increase, rather slowly at first, then quite rapidly throughout the pre-school period, and then more slowly as the child gets older. Vocabulary growth never ceases, since we all constantly learn new words and new usages of familiar words.

Average growth-rate of vocabulary

Child's age	Number of words acquired
Twelve months	3
Eighteen months	20
Two years	300
Three years	900/1000
Five years	2000

WORDS AND MEANING

One of the most striking characteristics of early language is that one word is used to mean a number of different things. These one-word sentences contain the same volume of meaning as adults would normally express in an entire sentence. The word 'Mama', for example, might mean 'Mama, I'm uncomfortable' or 'Mama, come here', etc. Development of sentences follows rapidly.

Stages in 'sentence' development

Age group	Sentence structure	For example
9–18 mths	One-element sentence	'Dada'; 'bye bye'
18–24 mths	Two-element sentences	'Dada gone'
2–2½ yrs	Three-element sentences	'Daddy kick ball'
2½–3 yrs	Increase in both length and structure	'Where my teddy gone?'
3–3½ yrs	Sentence + clause	'John gone into garden and he fell*ed* over'
3½–4½ yrs	Still some errors but use of pronouns, auxiliary verbs, irregular verbs, etc.	her/him/me/she/he is going, was doing, fell, caught, etc.
4½	Sentences complete, with few errors	

HOW YOU CAN HELP

Children's language development can be stimulated in many ways: this will also help later when they are learning reading and spelling.

- Talk and sing to your baby, from the beginning.

- Name the things you come across in your everyday interactions with your child, for example, name each item of clothes as you dress him in the morning, tell him what foods he is eating at mealtimes, what toys he is playing with, what is happening at bathtime, etc. Words must be heard a number of times before they will be used. When the child is using a number of nouns, introduce verbs, and have the child do the actions — jump, walk, etc. Speak slowly and clearly and keep it simple.

- Read stories to your child, and eventually encourage him to fill in parts of the stories. Ask questions about the stories.

- Nursery rhymes recited in unison will help to develop rhythm and rhyming of words.

- Engage your child in rhythmic activities, such as clapping, stamping, and generally moving to music.

- Play word games, for example 'I Spy'.

- Help him to join single words together to make one word, for example 'bus' and 'stop', and likewise to break up single words like 'pancake' to make two or more words.

- Practise rhyming words, for example, 'What word sounds like "man"?', etc.

SPEECH AND LANGUAGE DISORDERS

Some children will have normal speech and language development but will move through the stages at a slower rate. However, approximately 3 per cent of children will require the help of a speech and language therapist (SLT) if they are to acquire normal communication skills.

A child who has a speech disorder may have an articulation problem (difficulty in producing the normal sounds of speech) or he may have difficulty understanding words or forming words in his brain. Some children have both types of difficulty. Sometimes the disorder is the result of another problem, such as hearing loss, mental handicap, cleft palate or cerebral palsy.

Articulation problems are the most common. The child's speech may be unintelligible, except perhaps to his family. A small percentage of these difficulties will be caused by physical defects such as cleft palate, poor movement of the tongue or malaligned teeth (eg a gap between the upper and lower teeth, which may have been caused by extensive thumb-sucking or prolonged use of a soother). However, the majority of children with articulation difficulties have no such problem.

Common pronunciation problems include difficulties with the 'S' sound, so that the child may say 'tun' or 'thun' for 'sun', or he may pronounce his 'R's as 'W's, for instance 'wabbit' or 'wunning'. He may leave off the beginning or the end of a word. These children normally have no difficulty detecting errors in someone else's speech, but fail to be aware of their own errors. They cannot say what they want to say. Thus the following exchange can take place:

Child: Me play with the tat.
Adult: It's not a tat it's a cat.
Child: But I said tat.

Young children listening to tape recordings of their own speech have been heard to say, 'That girl is talking tunny!'

What should parents do?

Many children will grow out of their articulation problem with a little sympathetic help from their parents.

Do *not* correct the child. This will only serve to make the child conscious of his failure to meet your expectations.

Do say the word correctly and distinctly after the child, and build up a greater awareness of the sound. For example:

Child: John do to tool.
Adult: Yes! John goes to school.

When the child reaches the stage of being able to produce all his sounds but still has difficulty when two consonants come together, it can help to split the word and have him imitate you, for example:

Play: p-lay
School: s-chool
Blue: b-lue.

A far greater number of boys than girls will have difficulties in acquiring their sound system: a ratio of 4:1 is often given. There is often a family history of speech problems.

Children who have problems with sound-making often have other difficulties that are not so obvious. They may have difficulty in comprehending and using the grammatical structures of their language, especially when these structures become more complex. They are also very much at risk of developing problems with written language later on — with reading, spelling, formulating sentences, etc. This applies even to those children whose articulation problem seemed minimal and did not need speech or language therapy. The association between speech sounds, grammar and written language is based on the fact that they all deal with the structure of language, as opposed to vocabulary and semantics, which deal with the meaning of language.

LANGUAGE DIFFICULTIES

Children may have difficulties at any level of language acquisition. A child who can hear ordinary sounds around the house but who cannot understand language generally has quite a severe problem. Fortunately such children are rare; they will require intensive and specialised help.

Other children may have problems in using language, ranging from a slight difficulty with the more complex grammatical structures, to total absence of speech. In very severe cases the child may need to be taught a sign language in order to have some means of communication and to lessen his frustration until oral language is developed. The use of sign language will aid, rather than hinder, oral language development.

CHILDREN WITH MENTAL HANDICAP

Children with mental handicap experience a wide range of communication disorders. Some of their problems may result from additional disorders such as hearing loss, structural abnormalities, etc, while others will occur as a direct result of the mental handicap. It is important to realise that language development should be expected to occur in line with mental age and not actual age. Approximately 50 to 70 per cent of these children will require speech and language therapy.

Unfortunately, when it comes to speech and language therapy, there is a huge gap in the services provided in Ireland. While the majority of special schools have a full-time or sessional therapist, many more posts should be created to cope adequately with the requirements of all children in need of such therapy.

Speech and language therapy should form an integrated part of the daily management of these children, but it is important that parents know that one-to-one therapy is not always the ideal approach. Many children will benefit more from group therapy and/or the general work in the classroom, into which the therapist has an input. In addition to oral language, therapists will be involved in early feeding programmes (an area closely associated with speech) and in the teaching of sign language. Sign language may be the only means of communication for some severely handicapped children, or it may be the precursor to speech for others.

STUTTERING

This is probably the communication disorder that attracts most attention. The terms 'stuttering' and 'stammering' mean the same thing.

Everyone's speech has some pauses, repetitions and hesitations, but generally it is smooth, rhythmic and fluent. The label 'stuttering' is often applied when speech is characterised by repetitions of sounds or syllables, or by prolongations. Very often the label is applied to children when it should not be. Between the ages of two and six, many young children, in the course of developing their communication skills, go through a period of 'normal' non-fluency. When language develops late, this feature will also be seen at a later stage than is usual.

Causes

Stuttering tends to run in families, and is more common in boys. There has been much research into the cause, and many theories have been proposed, but there are as yet no conclusive answers as to why some children develop a stutter.

Some researchers believe that the source of the problem is in the brain, and is due to a delay in the formation of the myelin sheath that acts as insulation over the nerves in the brain. Other experts believe that the causes are psychological. The child may have been labelled a stutterer when he was going through a normal childhood phase of non-fluency, and this may have created anxiety and resulted in the child perceiving himself as a stutterer. Stuttering may occur because of a number of interacting factors, such as a family history of the condition, delay in processing speech, etc.

Another theory is that the factors that contribute to the continuation of the stutter are more important than the original cause, and that these need to be addressed.

Points for helping a child who stutters

- React unemotionally to the child's speech.
- Give the child plenty of time to speak.
- Build up the child's general self-confidence.
- Provide opportunities for the child to speak fluently, for example, saying nursery rhymes in unison *with* you, etc.
- Do not ask the child to recite 'party pieces'.
- Do not tell the child to stop and start again, or take a deep breath!
- Allow the child to complete sentences. Do not complete them for him.
- Put no pressure on speech and do not correct mispronunciations or grammar.

If your child's fluency doesn't improve and he moves from easy repetitions to tense utterances, and seems to avoid speaking, then he should be referred to a speech and language therapist.

VOICE DISORDERS

Disorders of voice in childhood form a small percentage of all childhood communication disorders. There are many factors that can cause disorders of the voice, but in all instances the child must be referred to an ear, nose and throat consultant before being referred to a speech and language therapist.

- Vocal abuse and vocal misuse, such as in screaming, yelling, shrieking: this often occurs when children commence team sports. Generally the resulting problem is temporary.
- Vocal nodules: these can result from consistent vocal abuse, and can occur on one or both vocal cords. If identified early, voice

therapy will help, but if the problem continues, surgical treatment followed by voice therapy will be required. Polyps (small tumours) may also occur from vocal abuse, sometimes after one instance of screaming, and again surgical treatment may be required along with voice therapy.

- Papillomata (wart-like growths that can grow anywhere in the airway) are a fairly common cause of hoarseness in children, and many require surgical treatment. Unfortunately there is a tendency for papillomata to recur.

- 'Puberphonia' is the term used to describe the persistence of an unnaturally high-pitched voice after the onset of puberty, and this problem will require referral to a speech and language therapist.

REFERRAL TO A SPEECH AND LANGUAGE THERAPIST

Your family doctor or your health centre can refer your child to a therapist. Speech and language therapists are located in community-care centres, hospitals and special schools. There are also a small number of therapists in private practice.

While there has been a large increase in the number of SLTs in the country in the last thirty years — from two in 1959 to 187 in 1992 — there is still a great shortfall. It is estimated that approximately five hundred more therapists are needed in Ireland to provide an adequate service for all the children who need therapy.

The therapist will begin by obtaining background information from the parents and by assessing the child to find out the exact nature of the problem. Sometimes additional referrals may be necessary, for example, to the psychologist, the audiologist (hearing specialist), etc. Therapy will be tailored to suit the individual child, and while in some instances he may attend in a group, in most cases therapy is on a one-to-one basis.

For the younger child, much of the therapy takes place in a play situation that is structured to deal with the language/speech problem. When the child is sufficiently mature to cooperate, the sessions will take on a more formal format, and the child will be required to carry out various exercises and procedures. Increasingly, computer-based instrumentation is becoming available for use both in assessment and therapy.

A parent will normally be present at the therapy sessions, which usually happen once a week, for several months or years. The sessions are only part of the therapy, and the work must be continued at home, with the parent and child doing the exercises together. This homework is essential if progress is to take place. The child also needs opportunities to put newly acquired skills into practice in a natural environment.

Sometimes the child will only need to attend a clinic at irregular intervals, following initial assessment and diagnosis. During these follow-up visits parents are advised on how to deal with the problem, and the child's progress is monitored until either normal communication is achieved or the child reaches his potential.

Children who have severe or multiple problems will require therapy sessions every day for a long period. The number of children with such severe language disorders is very small, but their needs are long term and cannot be met within the normal clinical setting. Their difficulties in language have repercussions in their total educational progress and social adjustment.

In recent years several language units have been established in Ireland, where the child attends on a daily basis and receives intensive therapy. Many more such units are required throughout the country, and at the present time there is a particular need for placements for the older children with language disorders, at both primary and secondary school levels.

Useful address

The Irish Association of Speech and Language Therapists, PO Box 1344, Dublin 4.

———————————————

Sr Marie de Montfort PhD, M Phil, FCSLT, DTST is Director of the School of Clinical Speech and Language Studies in Trinity College Dublin and President of the International Association of Logopedics and Phoniatrics.

TEETH

DR LIAM CONVERY

Children today have better teeth, fewer cavities, and are less afraid of going to the dentist. In general they have healthier diets, and fluoride in drinking water has had a dramatic effect on reducing tooth decay.

Good dental and oral health begins in childhood. Consultant paediatric dentist Dr Liam Convery explains how parents can help their children to have nice-looking teeth and healthy gums, and to preserve their smiles for life.

Parents are encouraged to bring children to see their dentist from about the age of three, so that preventive advice can be given from the outset. By going to the dentist at an early age, the first experience will be a pleasant one, and hopefully it will prevent the need for fillings, thereby reducing the costs of dentistry for their lifetime. Parents have to help children to clean their teeth and look after them, but they should encourage the child, and particularly the young adult, to assume responsibility for prevention as soon as possible. Good oral hygiene is only one aspect of general body hygiene, and good habits should be established early in life.

Prevention of dental disease and maintenance of oral health in children is based on the principle of avoiding sweets and sugary foods between meals, brushing with a fluoride toothpaste at least twice a day, and ensuring that children have sufficient fluoride in their drinking water.

TOOTH ERUPTION

The primary teeth (baby teeth) erupt at about six months of age. Usually the two lower front teeth erupt first, and within the first two years of life all twenty of the primary teeth have erupted. It is important to keep these teeth free from decay until they are shed naturally to allow the permanent teeth to succeed them.

The first permanent teeth start to erupt at six years of age. As the jaw grows and develops, more room is created for the bigger, stronger, permanent teeth. By the age of twelve or thirteen, all primary teeth should be gone, and twenty-eight of the thirty-two permanent teeth should have erupted. The four wisdom teeth erupt in the late teens, but they may be impacted (there may not be enough room for them to erupt) and sometimes they become infected. In most cases they eventually erupt, but often impacted wisdom teeth need to be removed. This can be more difficult than the normal extraction and your dentist will advise you.

TEETHING

In most cases, eruption of teeth causes no distress to the child, and parents are not aware that it is happening. Sometimes, however, there is local irritation, which is usually minor but may occasionally be severe enough to interfere with the child's sleep. You may see redness and swelling of the gum where the tooth is coming in, and the cheek may be flushed and red, with an increased flow of saliva leading to drooling. In more severe cases, the baby may be irritable, with loss of appetite and a disturbed sleep pattern. Teething has been blamed for many ailments, but there is little scientific evidence to support most of these associations. Parents often suffer more anxiety than the infant during teething!

The soreness may be temporarily relieved if the baby bites on a teething ring, particularly one that can be put in the fridge to chill. Hard rusks or biscuits can serve the same function, but they quickly become soft and may contain sugar or sweeteners. Teething gels such as Bonjela (sugar-free) contain local anaesthetic agents, but they can be very difficult to apply satisfactorily to a gum that is flooded with saliva, so it may be better to give the baby some liquid pain-killer, such as Calpol (sugar-free). These medications contain powerful drugs, so it is important that you do not exceed the stated dose, particularly with infants.

DENTAL DECAY

When we eat sugary food, an acid is formed in the mouth which attacks the enamel of the teeth for about thirty minutes and causes decay. The teeth can withstand up to four acid attacks a day, but when a child is snacking on sweet things continually, the teeth never get a chance to recover because they are constantly bathed in acid.

A quarter of all eight-year-olds and almost three quarters of all twelve-year-olds have cavities. There is one very obvious reason for this — sugar. It comes in a lot of different forms, not just in the obvious culprits like sweets, ice cream, biscuits, cakes, fizzy drinks and squashes, but also in most processed foods such as baked beans, tinned spaghetti and tomato ketchup.

You don't have to cut sweet things out of the diet completely, just control the number of times they are eaten. For instance, if a child has a packet of sweets, it is better that she finishes them at one go rather than spreading them out over the whole day. Try to discourage the habit of snacking between meals.

Brushing with a fluoride toothpaste helps the fight against decay, and this is particularly important in those parts of the country where there may be no fluoride in the water. Use a small amount of toothpaste — the size of a pea. Make sure that younger children do not swallow the toothpaste. Have them spit it out, but do not rinse immediately. If the fluoride is to have any effect it needs to be left in contact with the teeth for at least a minute.

The teeth should be brushed at least twice every day, and one of these brushings should be very thorough. We tend to miss the same places each time we brush, so be careful to clean all parts of all of the teeth. It will take about two or three minutes to remove the sticky dental plaque that collects on our teeth every day. Until a child is about eight, she will not have sufficient skill to do this properly for herself, so the parent should brush the child's teeth for her. You can use disclosing tablets occasionally, available from your pharmacist, to see how good the brushing technique is. Encouragement is better than nagging!

Baby bottles and decay

It is very distressing for everyone involved when a three or four-year-old child comes to the dentist with toothache as a result of extensive decay, particularly of the front teeth. This occurs when parents allow the child to hold the feeding bottle in her mouth for long periods of time, especially when she is sleeping. The situation is made worse if the baby's feed contains sugar. The infant's teeth are then bathed constantly in acid, and decay is rapid and inevitable.

This distressful and painful condition is totally preventable with a few simple precautions:

- Never let your child sleep with a bottle in her mouth.

- Don't allow your child to feed over prolonged periods.

- Don't put sugary drinks in your baby's bottle.

- Give your baby milk, water or unsweetened diluted fruit juices to drink. But remember, even unsweetened fruit juices have their own natural sugars, and these too can be harmful.

- Stop bottlefeeding when your child is a year old.

- Don't dip your baby's soother in sugar, honey or jam.

- Start brushing your child's teeth as soon as they erupt.

- Remember: 'Children should be fed and put to bed, NOT put to bed and fed'.

Fluoride

Fluoride makes tooth enamel harder and more resistant to decay. It also helps to repair and reverse the early stages of decay. Fluoride was first put into Irish drinking water twenty-five years ago, and since then the condition of our children's teeth has improved significantly. Fluoride in toothpaste has also had a dramatic effect in reducing decay. The rate of decay increases especially as children get older.

Fissure-sealing

Fissure-sealing can give extra protection to the biting surfaces of the teeth, and particularly to those children who are susceptible to decay. A clear plastic coating is placed in the fissure (groove) of the permanent molars (back teeth). Sealing the fissure prevents cavities from developing. The procedure is quick and painless, and usually protects the teeth for about five years. It should be done when the child is about six, after her first four permanent molars erupt, and again at twelve when the second group of permanent molars arrives.

The sick child

Parents are advised to give a sick child plenty of fluids — but they should always avoid sweet, sugary drinks. During an illness a child may become dehydrated because of sweating, and the mouth will be dry due to a great reduction in saliva. Saliva protects our teeth, gums and the lining of our mouth. If we add sweet, sugary drinks to the problem of a dry mouth, then we are almost certainly promoting tooth decay. Avoid treats that contain sugar at all times, but particularly during illness.

CHILDREN WITH PHYSICAL DISABILITIES AND/OR MEDICAL PROBLEMS

It is important not to forget the health of the mouth in children who have physical disabilities or medical problems.

It can be critically important for children with heart problems to have clean, healthy teeth and gums because they are at risk of infection from bacteria in the mouth, which can be linked to a potentially fatal condition — endocarditis. Children with damaged heart valves and some other related heart conditions may require antibiotics before certain dental procedures so as to protect their heart valves from bacteria released into the body during dental surgery. Prevention is very important for these children.

The child with Down's Syndrome is particularly susceptible to gum disease, and again, great care should be taken to encourage and promote healthy teeth and gums. Unfortunately, there is a natural tendency for the relatives of children who have long-term medical illness or physical or mental disability to bring them treats such as sweets, ice cream and sugary soft drinks.

Children who require long-term medication should be protected from having to take medicine in a syrup. Many of these syrups are made of flavoured sugar, and it is important to ask your chemist for an alternative form of medicine that does not contain sugar.

Children with physical disabilities may need extra help. There are special aids available to help physically disabled people carry out effective oral hygiene; ask the dentist or dental hygienist for advice.

STAINED TEETH

Teeth can be stained for a variety of reasons. Superficial stain can be due to certain mouth-washes (such as Corsodyl). Teeth can also be stained by an excessive amount of fluoride; this can be seen as white spots of varying degrees of severity on the teeth (mottling). A tooth that has been damaged in an accident may go black because the nerve inside the tooth loses its blood supply, causing the whole tooth to discolour. There are also developmental defects of the enamel parts of the tooth that can lead to serious malformation and staining of teeth. If your child's teeth are stained, ask your dentist for advice. There are several different treatments available, for example, bleaching, coating the teeth, veneers, capping (crowning), etc.

DAMAGE TO TEETH AND RESTORATIONS

Children's teeth can be damaged very easily during normal play. After an accident where the tooth has received a heavy blow, it will be sore for a while, and the nerve may die. If this happens, the tooth begins to darken, and may develop an abscess. If a front tooth is chipped, it can be built up again with a white filling material.

When a tooth is chipped, depending on the amount of tooth broken, the pulp may be exposed. It will appear as a red spot in the broken surface of the tooth, and will be exquisitely tender because it is a collection of exposed nerve endings. Telephone your dentist immediately and try to get an appointment straight away. If, as frequently happens, it is a newly erupted tooth whose roots have not fully formed, it is essential that treatment starts as soon as possible to save the nerve so that the growing root is allowed to complete its development. This may take several years. A broken mature tooth may need to have the pulp or nerve removed from it after an accident, and a root filling performed.

If a permanent tooth has been knocked out, go back to where the accident happened and find it, then pick it up without touching the root. There are live cells on the root of the tooth that will die after about ten minutes, so you need to move quickly to keep them alive. These cells are very important in the healing process. Don't touch the root, don't dry it, and don't try to sterilise it. If the tooth needs to be washed, don't put it anywhere near tap water, but wash it in milk from a freshly opened carton or bottle, or with some saline solution (the type you might use with contact lenses). Make sure you are holding the tooth the right way round, and push it back up into the socket. This might be a bit painful, but it should go right in on the first attempt. Get the child to bite firmly on a pad of tissues or cotton wool to hold the tooth in place. If the tooth won't go in straight away, put it into a container of fresh milk or saline solution. Or if the child is old enough not to swallow it, you can put the tooth into the pouch of her cheek to keep it safe and clean. Then go to the dentist immediately. The dentist may put a splint on the tooth and, if all goes well, the splint can be removed in a couple of weeks. Remember, if you want to save your child's tooth, move quickly. The first ten minutes are vital. As always, prevention is better; make sure that your child wears a mouthguard in all contact sports. A mouthguard made and fitted by a dentist is far more effective than one bought over the counter.

ORTHODONTICS

Orthodontics is the straightening of crooked teeth. It deals with a wide spectrum of problems, from the simple movement of a single tooth to complex rearrangement of all the teeth, including major jaw surgery.

Teeth move naturally as part of normal development, but they can also be moved artificially by the use of wires either directly attached to the teeth ('train tracks') or as finger springs on a removable plate. Light, continuous pressure is put on the teeth and they slowly shift position. The oral appliance may also be attached to a strap around the head.

There are a number of situations where orthodontic treatment may be required, for example, where there is a cleft palate (see below), where there is gross overcrowding of teeth, or very big spaces between the teeth, or where the child has very prominent, protruding teeth that are at risk from knocks and blows, and are spoiling the appearance. Occasionally, such anomalies can create speech problems and difficulties with cleaning.

The demand for orthodontic treatment comes mainly from a consideration of appearance. Before embarking on orthodontics, discuss the pros and cons with your dentist. Parents and children should realise that the process takes an average of eighteen months, requires many visits to the orthodontist, causes some discomfort, and is costly. During treatment, the child will need to take extra care with dental hygiene, because dental plaque (bacteria) accumulates very easily around the orthodontic appliances, and if proper care is not taken the child may end up with beautifully straight but decayed teeth, and gum disease. Children must take particular care to avoid sugars and eating between meals while wearing orthodontic appliances.

CLEFT LIP AND PALATE

About one in eight hundred babies is born with some form of cleft lip (harelip) or cleft palate (split in the roof of the mouth). This will be identified by the obstetrician or the paediatrician caring for the baby in the first few days, who will make the necessary referral for treatment. Infants with clefts often need special appliances for breast or bottle feeding.

The cleft between the mouth and the nasal airway presents great problems in sucking and breathing while feeding. Treatment will be provided by a plastic surgeon, together with an orthodontist, who can close the gap in the lip or palate. The first operation will usually take place when the infant is about three months old. Depending on the severity of the condition, the child may require a series of operations to close the palate and improve appearance. The orthodontist can reposition the bony arches that support the teeth so as to improve the position of the teeth, both before and after surgery.

Because teeth are so essential for a patient with cleft lip and palate, prevention of decay is of paramount importance. Loss of teeth can be very serious because the arches are malformed and every single tooth is important when attempting to restore normal function. Also, some teeth are critical as retainers for securing oral appliances which may be used to help seal off openings between the mouth and nasal airways in some patients with cleft palate.

SOME DO'S AND DON'TS

- Develop a regular, healthy feeding habit for your baby from the very outset, whether she is bottle fed or breast fed.

- Discourage all forms of snacking between meals, especially food containing sugar.

- If you live in an area where the water is not fluoridated, ask your dentist about fluoride supplements.

- Use a fluoride toothpaste.

- Encourage your child to wear a mouthguard when involved in any form of contact sport or activity.

- Help your child to brush her teeth up to the age of seven or eight — from then on she will be able to do it herself.

- Do not reward children with sweets.

- Do not bring presents of sweets to children, and particularly to those with long-term illness.

- Never refer to the dentist as a person to be afraid of.

- Do not wait for dental decay or toothache to occur before bringing your child to visit the dentist.

- Encourage, but don't nag, when promoting better health habits.

Useful address

The Cleft Lip and Palate Association of Ireland, 152 Ard na Mara, Malahide, Co Dublin Tel. (01) 8450234.
Irish Dental Health Foundation, Richview, Clonskea Road, Dublin 4. Tel. (01) 2830363.

Dr Liam Convery BDS, MScD is a senior lecturer/consultant in paediatric dentistry at the Dublin Dental Hospital and the School of Dental Science, Trinity College Dublin, and Consultant Paediatric Dentist to the National Children's Hospital, Harcourt Street, Dublin.

HEALTH RECORD CHART

Child's Name: _____   Weight at birth: _____

Date of Birth: _____   Height at birth: _____

HEIGHT AND WEIGHT

Age (date)	Height	Weight
_____	_____	_____
_____	_____	_____
_____	_____	_____
_____	_____	_____
_____	_____	_____
_____	_____	_____
_____	_____	_____
_____	_____	_____
_____	_____	_____
_____	_____	_____

IMMUNISATIONS

Immunisation	Date	Comments
BCG		
DTP/polio/HiB		
DTP/polio/HiB		
DTP/polio/HiB		
MMR		
DTP/polio		
MMR		
BCG		

ILLNESSES

Date	Problem	Treatment

DENTAL TREATMENT

Date	Problem	Treatment

EMERGENCY ADDRESSES/PHONE NUMBERS

Doctor: _____

Hospital: _____

Health centre: _____

Public health nurse:_____

Dentist: _____

RECOMMENDED READING

Carson, Dr Paul. *Coping Successfully With Your Child's Asthma.* Sheldon Press, London.
How to Cope With Your Child's Allergies. Sheldon Press, London.

Douglas, J and Richman, N. *My Child Won't Sleep.* Penguin, London, 1984.

Farmar, Anna. *Children's Last Days.* Town House, Dublin, 1992.

Gaffney, Maureen, Conway, Andy, Andrews, Paul, and Fitzgerald, Frances. *Parenting: A Handbook for Parents.* Town House, Dublin, 1991.

Hanssen, Maurice and Marsden, Jill. *E for Additives: the Complete E Number Guide.* Thorsons Publishers Ltd, 1984.

Hornsby, Bevé. *Before Alpha. Learning Games of the Under Fives.* Souvenir Press, 1989.

Illingworth, R. *The Normal Child.* (10th edition.) Churchill Livingstone, Edinburgh, 1991.

McMenamin, Dr Joe and O'Connor Bird, Mary. *Epilepsy: A Parent's Guide.* Brainwave (The Irish Epilepsy Association), 1993.

Tanner, J M. *Foetus Into Man.* (2nd edition.) Castlemead Publications, Ware, 1989.

LEAFLETS AND BROCHURES

Additive Decoder — pocket-size booklet on food additives. Stg £1.55, including P & P, from 'Foresight', 28 The Paddock, Surrey GU7 IXD, England.

Communication Needs (1989), available from The Irish Association of Speech and Language Therapists, PO Box 1344, Dublin 4.

The following leaflets are available free from the Health Promotion Unit, Dept of Health, Hawkins House, Hawkins Street, Dublin 2. Tel. (01) 6714711:
> *Food for Babies*
> *Play it Safe,* and other safety leaflets
> *Protect Your Child, Immunise*

Various publications and fact sheets on child safety are available from: The Child Accidents Prevention Trust, Fourth Floor, Clerks Court, 18-20 Farringdon Lane, London, ECIR 3AU. Tel. (071) 608 3838. Fax (071) 608 3674.

INDEX